# Cancer-Related Fatigue

T0075427

Joachim Weis • Markus Horneber

# Cancer-Related Fatigue

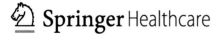
Springer Healthcare

Joachim Weis
Department of Psycho-Oncology
Tumor Biology Centre
Freiburg
Germany

Markus Horneber
Department of Oncology/Hematology
Paracelsus Medical University
Klinikum Nuernberg
Nuernberg
Germany

ISBN 978-1-907673-75-7          ISBN 978-1-907673-76-4     (eBook)
DOI 10.1007/978-1-907673-76-4
Springer Tarporley Heidelberg New York Dordrecht London

Library of Congress Control Number: 2014952681

Printed on acid-free paper

Springer is part of Springer Science+Business Media (www.springer.com)

# Contents

# Chapter 1
# Definition and Prevalence of Cancer-Related Fatigue

## 1.1 Introduction

Cancer-related fatigue (CrF) is among the most common sequelae precipitated by cancer and cancer treatments. It is severely undertreated and contributes to impaired functioning, decline in overall quality of life, and significant socioeconomic costs. Research supports that CrF is associated with shorter survival and increased mortality rates. According to epidemiological studies, more than 30 % of patients newly diagnosed with cancer will experience moderate-to-severe CRF in the first year after diagnosis. The more severe the symptoms of CrF, the more likely they are to persist or recur, even after cancer treatment has ceased or if the patient is in remission. Thus, assessment and treatment of CrF should be initiated early, with continuous monitoring in all patients diagnosed with cancer.

J. Weis, M. Horneber, *Cancer-Related Fatigue*,
DOI 10.1007/978-1-907673-76-4_1,
© Springer Healthcare 2015

## 1.2   Physiologic Fatigue

At the end of the 19th century, Angelo Mosso, a Professor of Physiology at the University of Turin, described the body's reaction to stress as:

> ...at first sight...an imperfection of our body, but is on the contrary, one of its most marvelous perfections. The fatigue increasing more rapidly than the amount of work done saves us from the injury which lesser sensibility would involve for the organism... [1].

Fatigue, exhaustion, and diminished physical and psychological performance are common physical reactions to stress and are connected with subjective perceptions and objective changes that can often be reversible and recede after rest or sleep. Depending on the type and intensity of the stress exposure, typical subjective perceptions include tiredness, heaviness of limbs, blurred vision, tinnitus, dyspnea, nausea, apathy towards external stimuli, or myalgias. Objective symptoms include muscular, neuropsychological, and metabolic changes including reduced muscle strength, tremor, diminished reflex responses, impaired coordination, diminished concentration, attention and memory problems, electrolyte abnormalities, lactate increase, and reduction of glycogen. Research over the last decade has shown that fatigue is part of complex self-regulation of physiological systems, the goal of which is to protect the body from harm. The central nervous system (CNS) uses the symptoms of fatigue and exhaustion, especially after physical exertion, as important regulators to ensure that an effort is stopped before it results in damage [2].

## 1.3   Pathologic Fatigue

Fatigue and increased fatigability are common reactions to non-pathological physical and psychological strain and stress but also occur as symptoms in almost every medical and psychiatric condition. Hence, persisting symptoms and signs of fatigue that are not relieved by sleep or physical rest may be an indication of a serious medical problem. Accordingly, many chronic conditions such as rheumatoid arthritis, cardio-vascular disease, and multiple sclerosis are also associated with fatigue. A meta-analysis by Lewis and Wessely reported that the odds ratios (ORs) for fatigue in chronic diseases (e.g., emphysema, asthma, heart failure, and arthritis) are between 1.9 and 2.9, and that the risk is even higher for psychiatric disorders (OR 3.0–6.0) [3]. Fatigue can occur as a concomi-tant symptom or, as in the case of depression, represent a primary symptom. It is quite possible that fatigue has more than one simultaneous cause, even when it is associated with a clear diagnosis [4].

## 1.4   Cancer-Related Fatigue

The syndrome of fatigue and exhaustion in cancer patients is described as CrF if it is not a manifestation of a pre-existing condition or disease and it is this term that will be used throughout the book. (Other terms such as cancer fatigue or cancer treatment-related fatigue are also used in clinical and research literature and patient educational material to describe the same condition). CrF is commonly defined as a self-recognized phenomenon that is subjective in nature and experienced as a feeling of tiredness or lack of energy that varies in degree, frequency, and duration, which is not proportional to physical activities, and not relieved by sleep or rest [5, 6]. Patients often describe CrF as an unusual feeling of exhaustion, weakness, or a loss of activity, with sequels to emotional and cognitive functions [5–8].

**Cancer-related fatigue is a distressing persistent sub-jective sense of physical, emotional, and cognitive tiredness or exhaustion related to cancer or cancer treatment that is not proportional to recent activity and interferes with usual functioning [5].**

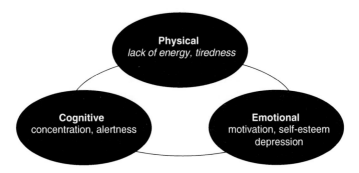

**Fig. 1.1** Multidimensional structure of cancer-related fatigue. This figure shows the three domains of the multidimensional model of cancer-related fatigue: physical, cognitive, and emotional

Clinical investigation into CrF primarily started in the 1970s as an interest of nursing and psychological researchers [9]. Since then, several studies have been published investigating the prevalence and associative factors of CrF in cancer patients, as well as suitable assessment strategies [7]. In most publications, CrF has been described not only as a physical symptom but as a multi-dimensional construct including physical, cognitive, and emotional dimensions [7]. The physical domain describes fatigue as a loss of ability to perform activities due to somatic symptoms of tiredness and loss of energy. The mental or cognitive dimension includes losses of concentration and attention, reduced alertness, and impairment in short-term memory. The emotional dimension covers symptoms such as loss of motivation, reduced self-esteem, and depressive feelings (Fig. 1.1).

## 1.5 Epidemiology and Prevalence Rates

CrF is one of the most common symptoms caused by cancer and therapies used to treat cancer (e.g., chemotherapy). For example, CrF may occur during or after medical treatment or as a long-term late effect some time after cessation of anti-cancer treatment. Based on several epidemiological studies, prevalence rates of CrF range from 59–100 % in patients with cancer [10, 11]. The differences in the various prevalence rates may be explained by the way that fatigue is assessed, as well as the fatigue criteria used.

During the last decade, studies have emphasized the complex problems faced by patients with cancer who experience CrF during or after treatment, underscoring how important an issue fatigue can be. Specifically, it was determined to affect significantly more patients, more often, than any other cancer-related symptom and had a more of an effect on the patient's quality of life than pain, nausea, or vomiting ($P < 0.0001$) [12]. The highest CrF prevalence rates were found as a direct side effect of a combination of medical therapies such as surgery, chemotherapy, radiotherapy, hormone therapy, and with the use of certain treatments such as hematopoietic stem cell transplantation or high-dose chemotherapy [10, 13–15]. A recent study showed that a majority of patients with cancer reported feeling fatigued at least once a week during treatment (Fig. 1.2) [16].

Fatigue during treatment has been found to be a risk factor for developing chronic CrF following treatment [17, 18]. CrF can persist or recur as a long-term sequelae for many years after treatment has ceased and may cause persistent functional impairment [19–21]. Depending on how it is assessed, CrF in long-term survivors occurs in approximately 25–35 % of patients [22]. It has been found that CrF rates are higher in certain tumors (e.g., pancreatic, breast, lymphoma) and that CrF is associated with shorter survival and increased mortality [23, 24].

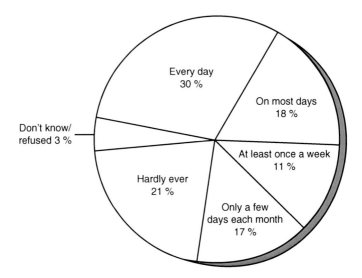

**Fig. 1.2** Prevalence of fatigue in patients with cancer. Three hundred and seventy nine patients with cancer were asked how often they felt fatigued while undergoing their most recent cancer treatment. Fatigue was defined as a feeling of debilitating tiredness or loss of energy. (Reproduced with permission from Curt et al. [16] ©Alphamed Press)

## 1.6  Clinical Manifestation

The clinical manifestation of CrF is multifaceted and the perceived problems and limitations affect patients in a highly individual manner [25]. In comparison with healthy individuals who experience fatigue as a 'normal' sensation that is associated with daily routine and activities, in patients with CrF, symptoms may appear suddenly or after minimal levels of exertion, leading to physical exhaustion, fatigue, weakness, and heaviness in the limbs. Many patients also complain of concentration and memory problems, feelings of apathy, and lack of drive [26]. Typically, the symptoms are not proportional to the preceding activities and after recovery periods or sleep, improvement may only occur for a short time, if at all [27].

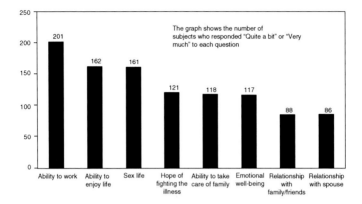

**Fig. 1.3** Effects of fatigue on activities of daily life. Patients with cancer (n = 538) were asked to what extent they felt that fatigue affected aspects of their life. (Reproduced with permission from Stone et al. [12] ©Wolters Kluwer)

Symptoms and signs of CrF can appear at any time during the course of cancer [28], including:

- as an early symptom before the diagnosis of cancer and then occurring again for a limited time after a course of chemotherapy ('rollercoaster');
- with slowly and steadily increasing intensity and persisting over a prolonged period during radiotherapy;
- as a symptom of relapse or progression; and/or
- persisting after completion of successful curative cancer therapy.

## 1.7  Impact of Fatigue

CrF often seriously impacts the quality of life of patients and affects daily activities, work, and family life (Fig. 1.3) [12, 16, 18, 29]. Ahlberg and colleagues found statistically significant negative correlations between fatigue and various domains of quality of life, including effects on physical, emotional, cognitive, social, sexual, and role functioning (ie, activities of daily living) [30]. They also showed further that physical and cognitive functioning remained highly negatively correlated with general fatigue over time [30]. For patients receiving palliative or end-of-life care, CrF can be associated with highly limited, or even loss of, body functions and a decline in overall quality of life [31].

CrF not only affects the individual patient but also the patient's partners and relatives [32]. Patients often report that persisting fatigue is not always understood by the people close to them and social conflicts can arise, which may result in further social withdrawal or isolation.

CrF can also have consequences on health expenditure, as patients presenting with CrF show a higher rate of physician counseling requests, private practitioner support, and use of other health services [12, 33]. CrF has also been shown to have a significant effect on employment and financial status. Curt et al. reported higher rates of sick leave, loss of work capacity, and forced changes to conditions of employment due to CrF in patients with breast cancer [29]. Moreover, CrF has been proven to be a negative predictor of the rate of work resumption after cancer treatment [34, 35].

# References

1. Mosso A. Fatigue. London: Allen and Unwin Ltd; 1905.
2. Noakes TD. Fatigue is a brain-derived emotion that regulates the exercise behavior to ensure the protection of whole body homeostasis. Front Physiol. 2012;3:82.
3. Lewis G, Wessely S. The epidemiology of fatigue: more questions than answers. J Epidemiol Community Health. 1992;46:92–7.
4. Wessely S. Chronic fatigue: symptom and syndrome. Ann Intern Med. 2001;134:838–43.
5. Wagner LI, Cella D. Fatigue and cancer: causes, prevalence and treatment approaches. Br J Cancer. 2004;91:822–8.
6. Henry DH, Viswanathan HN, Elkin EP, et al. Symptoms and treatment burden associated with cancer treatment: results from a cross-sectional survey in the U.S. Support Care Cancer. 2008;16:791–801.

7. National Comprehensive Cancer Network (NCCN). Clinical practice guidelines in oncology: cancer related fatigue. Version 1. 2014. www.nccn. org/professionals/physician_gls/pdf/fatigue.pdf. Accessed 25 September 2014.

8. Cella D, Davis K, Breitbart W, Curt G. Cancer related fatigue: prevalence of proposed diagnostic criteria in a United States Sample of cancer survivors. J Clin Oncol. 2001;19:3385–91.

9. Glaus A. Fatigue in patients with cancer: analysis and assessment. Heidelberg/Germany: Springer; 1998.

10. Irvine D, Vincent L, Graydon J, Bubela N, Thompson L. The prevalence and correlates of fatigue in patients receiving treatment with chemotherapy and radiotherapy. Cancer Nurs. 1994;17:367–78.

11. Morrow GR, Andrews PL, Hickok JT, et al. Fatigue associated with cancer and its treatment. Support Care Cancer. 2002;10:389–98.

12. Stone P, Richardson A, Ream E, et al. Cancer-related fatigue: inevitable, unimportant, and untreatable? Results of a multi-centre patient survey. Cancer Fatigue Forum. Ann Oncol. 2000;11:971–5.

13. Servaes P, Verhagen C, Bleijenberg G. Fatigue in cancer patients during and after treatment: prevalence, correlates and interventions. Eur J Cancer. 2002;38:27–43.

14. Neitzert C, Ritvo P, Dancey J, Weiser K, Murray C, Avery J. The psychosocial impact of bone marrow transplantation: a review of the literature. Bone Marrow Transplant. 1998;22:409–22.

15. Wettergren L, Langius A, Björkholm M, Björvell H. Physical and psychosocial functioning in patients undergoing autologous bone marrow transplantation – a prospective study. Bone Marrow Transplant. 1997; 20:497–502.

16. Curt GA, Breitbart W, Cella D, et al. Impact of cancer-related fatigue on the lives of patients: new findings from the fatigue coalition. Oncologist. 2000;5:353–60.

17. Kuhnt S, Ehrensperger C, Singer S, et al. Prädiktoren tumorassoziierter Fatigue. Psychotherapeut. 2011;56:216–23.

18. Andrykowski MA, Donovan KA, Laronga C, Jacobsen PB. Prevalence, predictors, and characteristics of off-treatment fatigue in breast cancer survivors. Cancer 2010; 116:5740–8.

19. Rueffer JU, Flechtner H, Tralls P, et al. Fatigue in long-term survivors of Hodgkin's lymphoma; a report from the German Hodgkin Lymphoma Study Group (GHSG). Eur J Cancer. 2003;39:2179–86.

20. Berglund G, Boland C, Fornandes T, et al. Late effects of adjuvant chemotherapy and postoperative radiotherapy on quality of life among breast cancer patients. Eur J Cancer. 1991;27:1075–81.

21. Bower J, Ganz P, Desmond K, Rowland J, Meyerowitz B, Belin R. Fatigue in breast cancer survivors: occurrence, correlates, an impact of quality of life. J Clin Oncol. 2000;18:743–53.

22. Servaes P, van der Werf S, Prins J, Verhagen S, Bleijenberg G. Fatigue in disease-free cancer patients compared with fatigue in patients with chronic fatigue syndrome. Support Care Cancer. 2001;9:11–7.
23. Gotay CC, Kawamoto CT, Bottomley A, Efficace F, et al. The prognostic significance of patient-reported outcomes in cancer clinical trials. J Clin Oncol. 2008;26:1355–63.
24. Montazeri A. Quality of life data as prognostic indicators of survival in cancer patients: an overview of the literature from 1982 to 2008. Health Qual Life Outcomes. 2009;7:102.
25. Scott JA, Lasch KE, Barsevick AM, Piault-Louis E. Patients' experiences with cancer-related fatigue: a review and synthesis of qualitative research. Oncol Nurs Forum. 2011;38:E191–203.
26. Glaus A, Crow R, Hammond S. A qualitative study to explore the concept of fatigue/tiredness in cancer patients and in healthy individuals. Eur J Cancer Care (Engl). 1996;5(2 suppl):8–23.
27. Servaes P, Gielissen MF, Verhagen S, Bleijenberg G. The course of severe fatigue in disease-free breast cancer patients: a longitudinal study. Psychooncology. 2007;16:787–95.
28. Bruera E. Cancer-related fatigue: a multidimensional syndrome. J Support Oncol. 2010;8:175–6.
29. Smith SK, Herndon JE, Lyerly HK, et al. Correlates of quality of life-related outcomes in breast cancer patients participating in the Pathfinders pilot study. Psychooncology. 2011;20:559–64.
30. Ahlberg K, Ekman T, Gaston-Johansson F. Fatigue, psychological distress, coping resources, and functional status during radiotherapy for uterine cancer. Oncol Nurs Forum. 2005;32:633–40.
31. Olson K, Krawchuk A, Quddusi T. Fatigue in individuals with advanced cancer in active treatment and palliative settings. Cancer Nurs. 2007;30:E1–10.
32. Oktay JS, Bellin MH, Scarvalone S, Appling S, Helzlsouer KJ. Managing the impact of posttreatment fatigue on the family: breast cancer survivors share their experiences. Fam Syst Health. 2011;29:127–37.
33. Servaes P, Verhagen S, Schreuder HW, et al. Fatigue after treatment for malignant and benign bone and soft tissue tumors. J Pain Symptom Manage. 2003;26:1113–22.
34. Spelten ER, Verbeek JH, Uitterhoeve AL, et al. Cancer, fatigue and the return of patients to work – a prospective cohort study. Eur J Cancer. 2003;39:1562–7.
35. Tiedtke C, de Rijk A, Dierckx de Casterle B, Christiaens MR, Donceel P. Experiences and concerns about 'returning to work' for women breast cancer survivors: a literature review. Psychooncology. 2010;19:677–83.

# Chapter 2
# Etiology and Pathogenesis of Cancer-Related Fatigue

## 2.1 Introduction

Attempts to explain the etiology and pathogenesis of cancer-related fatigue (CrF) assume complex and multicausal processes in which somatic, emotional, and cognitive factors interact and ultimately lead to fatigue and a reduction in performance. Thus, it is assumed that one or more factors of each of these categories are conditional for the development of CrF [1, 2]. With CrF, these processes can have tumor-related causes or could be the result of the cancer therapy, as well as being influenced by genetic predisposition, epigenetic changes, concomitant somatic or mental disorders, and environmental factors [1, 2]. However, despite the high prevalence of CrF, the underlying mechanisms remain poorly understood.

## 2.2 Symptom Clustering and Inflammation

CrF often co-occurs with other symptoms such as mood disorders, sleep disturbances, and other cognitive dysfunctions which follow a similar time course in relation to treatment or disease

J. Weis, M. Horneber, *Cancer-Related Fatigue*,
DOI 10.1007/978-1-907673-76-4_2,
© Springer Healthcare 2015

and have been designated as 'symptom clusters' [3]. There is growing evidence that such symptom clusters share similar pathogenic mechanisms and several lines of evidence point to the fact that CrF, as part of such a symptom cluster, is central in origin and that inflammation appears to be the mediating process between the possible causes and the symptoms [4, 5].

In considering the relationship between immunological factors and CrF, a meta-analysis by Saligan and colleagues found that patients with CrF had elevated levels of markers for systemic inflammation (e.g., C-reactive protein [CRP], polymorphonuclear leukocytes), CD4+ T cells, proinflammatory cytokines (interleukin [IL]-6, IL-1-β), as well as IL-1 receptor antagonists and soluble TNF receptor II [6]. It is also known that chemotherapy and radiotherapy lead to an increase of numerous proinflammatory cytokines and chemokines [7–11]. For example, the results of a recent longitudinal study demonstrated a clear link between CrF and increased soluble TNF receptor I and IL-6 levels during chemoradiation therapy for colorectal and esophageal cancer [12].

## 2.2.1   Sickness Behavior Syndrome

In 2003, Cleeland et al. reported a clinical similarity between the symptoms expressed by cancer patients and the physiologic components of sickness behavior syndrome (SBS) elicited by infection and acute inflammation [13]. SBS is characterized by fever, general fatigue, anorexia (loss of appetite), insomnia, decrease in activity, and cognitive impairment, mirroring symptoms produced by cancers and cancer treatments; there is growing awareness that common biologic mechanisms may underlie or contribute to at least some of those symptoms. Recent findings have begun to unravel a number of interesting inflammatory and immunological explanations that suggest CrF and SBS are interrelated, yet distinct, conditions [4, 14]. As a

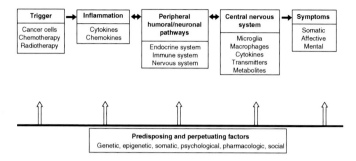

**Fig. 2.1** Pathophysiological model of the development of cancer-related fatigue as immune-induced sickness behavior. Cellular damage leads to the formation of proinflammatory cyto- and chemokines by immunocompetent cells. The inflammation is routed to the central nervous system (CNS) through various pathways, and here, the peripheral terminals of sensory neurons and the brain-resident perivascular macrophages and microglial cells play a central role in immune-to-brain signaling. Within the CNS, changes in the levels of cytokines, transmitters, and metabolites result. (Adapted with permission from Dantzer et al. [4] ©Elsevier)

common pathogenetic principle of CrF and SBS, Dantzer et al. and Bower and Lamkin suggested a cause-effect chain that emanates from a cellular and humoral immune response as a result of stressors such as chemotherapeutic agents or ionizing radiation (Fig. 2.1). This, in turn, causes neuronal, endocrine, immunological, and metabolic changes, leading to alterations of cytokines, prostaglandins, neurotransmitters, and their metabolites within the CNS (Fig. 2.1) [4, 14].

In radiation therapy, for example, reactive oxygen and nitrogen species are released which mediate detrimental effects not only to irradiated cancer cells but also to non-targeted cells causing short- and long-term 'bystander effects' through cytokine stimulation [9]. Current data suggest that the inflammatory response from bystander cells can persist and may trigger treatment-related SBS [15].

## 2.2.2  Fatigue and the Central Nervous System

CrF should be understood as a dysregulation of the CNS leading to the symptoms of fatigue and causing neuroendocrine and metabolic changes in the organism in its wake. Manifestations of dysregulation and subsequent changes in patients with CrF include, for example:

- disorders of the diurnal secretion of cortisol [16], melatonin [17], body temperature [18], circulating leukocytes and cytokines [19], and sleep-wake cycles [20–22];
- decreased numbers of serotonin transporters (5-HTT) in the cingulate gyrus and polymorphisms in the serotonin transporter gene [23, 24]; and
- "central activation failure" and changes in cortical and spinal centers of the sensorimotor system as a cause of reduced muscular performance [25, 26].

## 2.2.3  Genetic Factors

The presence of gene polymorphisms for regulatory proteins involved in oxidative phosphorylation, signal transduction in B cells, the expression of proinflammatory cytokines, and catecholamine metabolism have been found in patients with CrF. These poylmorphisms may possibly influence the development, severity, and the progress of CrF [27, 28]. For example, current research suggests that genetic factors such as the Val158Met polymorphism of the catechol-O-methyltransferase (COMT) gene might play a distinct role in the manifestation of CRF [29].

Although recent research in to CrF and associated symptom clusters have produced many exciting new findings and possible perspectives, Dantzer et al. notes that comprehension of the mechanisms underlying the development of treatment-related symptom clusters remains limited. However, there is growing awareness of the common biological mechanisms (e.g., inflammatory response produced by disease or treatment, endocrine impairment, hematopoietic dysfunction) that may cause or contribute to some of these symptoms concurrently [4].

# References

1. Bruera E. Cancer-related fatigue: a multidimensional syndrome. J Support Oncol. 2010;8:175–6.
2. Barsevick A, Frost M, Zwinderman A, Hall P, Halyard M. I'm so tired: biological and genetic mechanisms of cancer-related fatigue. Qual Life Res. 2010;19:1419–27.
3. Kenne Sarenmalm E, Browall M, Gaston-Johansson F. Symptom burden clusters: a challenge for targeted symptom management. A longitudinal study examining symptom burden clusters in breast cancer. J Pain Symptom Manage. 2014;47:731–41.
4. Dantzer R, Meagher MW, Cleeland CS. Translational approaches to treatment-induced symptoms in cancer patients. Nat Rev Clin Oncol. 2012;9:414–26.
5. Wood LJ, Weymann K. Inflammation and neural signaling: etiologic mechanisms of the cancer treatment-related symptom cluster. Curr Opin Support Palliat Care. 2013;7:54–9.
6. Saligan LN, Kim HS. A systematic review of the association between immunogenomic markers and cancer-related fatigue. Brain Behav Immun. 2012;26:830–48.
7. Brode S, Cooke A. Immune-potentiating effects of the chemotherapeutic drug cyclophosphamide. Crit Rev Immunol. 2008;28:109–26.
8. Elsea CR, Roberts DA, Wood LJ, et al. Inhibition of p38 MAPK suppresses inflammatory cytokine induction by etoposide, 5-fluorouracil, and doxorubicin without affecting tumoricidal activity. PLoS One. 2008;3:e2355.
9. Hei TK, Zhou H, Chai Y, et al. Radiation induced non-targeted response: mechanism and potential clinical implications. Curr Mol Pharmacol. 2011;4:96–105.
10. Mahoney SE, Davis JM, Murphy EA, et al. Effects of 5-fluorouracil chemotherapy on fatigue: role of MCP-1. Brain Behav Immun. 2013; 27:155–61.

11. Tsavaris N, Kosmas C, Vadiaka M, et al. Immune changes in patients with advanced breast cancer undergoing chemotherapy with taxanes. Br J Cancer. 2002;87:21–7.

12. Wang XS, Williams LA, Krishnan S, et al. Serum sTNF-R1, IL-6, and the development of fatigue in patients with gastrointestinal cancer undergoing chemoradiation therapy. Brain Behav Immun. 2012;26: 699–705.

13. Cleeland CS, Bennett GJ, Dantzer R, et al. Are the symptoms of cancer and cancer treatment due to a shared biologic mechanism? A cytokineimmunologic model of cancer symptoms. Cancer. 2003;97:2919–25.

14. Bower JE, Lamkin DM. Inflammation and cancer-related fatigue: mechanisms, contributing factors, and treatment implications. Brain Behav Immun. 2012;30(suppl):48–57.

15. Hsiao CP, Araneta M, Wang XM, Saligan LN. The association of IFI27 expression and fatigue intensification during localized radiation therapy: implication of a para-inflammatory bystander response. Int J Mol Sci. 2013;14:16943–57.

16. Weinrib AZ, Sephton SE, Degeest K, et al. Diurnal cortisol dysregulation, functional disability, and depression in women with ovarian cancer. Cancer. 2010;116:4410–9.

17. Mazzoccoli G, Carughi S, De CA, et al. Neuroendocrine alterations in lung cancer patients. Neuro Endocrinol Lett. 2003;24:77–82.

18. Sephton S, Spiegel D. Circadian disruption in cancer: a neuroendocrine-immune pathway from stress to disease? Brain Behav Immun. 2003;17: 321–8.

19. Innominato PF, Mormont MC, Rich TA, et al. Circadian disruption, fatigue, and anorexia clustering in advanced cancer patients: implications for innovative therapeutic approaches. Integr Cancer Ther. 2009; 8:361–70.

20. Rich TA. Symptom clusters in cancer patients and their relation to EGFR ligand modulation of the circadian axis. J Support Oncol. 2007; 5:167–74.

21. Rumble ME, Keefe FJ, Edinger JD, et al. Contribution of cancer symptoms, dysfunctional sleep related thoughts, and sleep inhibitory behaviors to the insomnia process in breast cancer survivors: a daily process analysis. Sleep. 2010;33:1501–9.

22. Jim HS, Small B, Faul LA, et al. Fatigue, depression, sleep, and activity during chemotherapy: daily and intraday variation and relationships among symptom changes. Ann Behav Med. 2011;42:321–33.

23. Yamamoto S, Ouchi Y, Onoe H, et al. Reduction of serotonin transporters of patients with chronic fatigue syndrome. Neuroreport. 2004;15:2571–4.
24. Narita M, Nishigami N, Narita N, et al. Association between serotonin transporter gene polymorphism and chronic fatigue syndrome. Biochem Biophys Res Commun. 2003;311:264–6.
25. Kisiel-Sajewicz K, Davis MP, Siemionow V. Lack of muscle contractile property changes at the time of perceived physical exhaustion suggests central mechanisms contributing to early motor task failure in patients with cancer-related fatigue. J Pain Symptom Manage. 2012;44:351–61.
26. Yavuzsen T, Davis MP, Ranganathan VK, et al. Cancer-related fatigue: central or peripheral? J Pain Symptom Manage. 2009;38:587–96.
27. Bower JE, Ganz PA, Irwin MR, et al. Cytokine genetic variations and fatigue among patients with breast cancer. J Clin Oncol. 2013;31: 1656–61.
28. Reinertsen KV, Grenaker Alnæs GI, et al. Fatigued breast cancer survivors and gene polymorphisms in the inflammatory pathway. Brain Behav Immun. 2011;25:1376–83.
29. Fernandez-de-Las-Penas C, et al. Breast Cancer Res Treat 2012;133: 405–12.

# Chapter 3
# Diagnosis and Assessment

## 3.1 Introduction

Assessment and clinical diagnosis of cancer-related fatigue (CrF) is an important task for health care professionals that provide cancer care and is a prerequisite for determining proper strategies for the management of CrF in the individual patient.

Due to the multifactorial disease etiologies, diagnosis and assessment of CrF is a major challenge. However, a comprehensive assessment can provide insight into underlying causal factors, which in turn could indicate appropriate treatment strategies.

Although aims of assessment of CrF in the clinical setting differ from that in research, both rely on self-report measures because fatigue is primarily a subjectively experienced cluster of symptoms. Multidimensional questionnaires provide a sophisticated ways of assessing CrF but they are often too time-consuming in clinical practice and burdensome for the patient. Current guidelines propose a structured approach for the clinical assessment of CrF, including screening for the presence and severity of CrF during the preliminary clinical encounter, and, if the screening reveals moderate or severe CrF, a focused history,

J. Weis, M. Horneber, *Cancer-Related Fatigue*,
DOI 10.1007/978-1-907673-76-4_3,
© Springer Healthcare 2015

thorough physical examination, and targeted laboratory investigations.

## 3.2  Diagnostic Criteria

CrF is commonly defined as a symptom, rather than a stand-alone disease. For example, in the World Health Organization's *International Classification of Diseases* (ICD), fatigue is not discussed alongside other psychosomatic or somatization disorders such as chronic fatigue syndrome (CFS) or neurasthenia [1]. Although CrF is distinguished from CFS and other types of fatigue, there are indeed some similarities and overlaps with respect to phenomenology and theoretical explanations [2]. For example, if symptoms and signs of fatigue last for an extended period of time without a defined cause, and if other defined criteria are present, the patient should be diagnosed with CFS [3, 4]. This distinction is especially important to consider for fatigue in long-term cancer survivors, especially those who are either cured (solid tumors) or in complete remission (without any signs of tumor activity) for many years. In those cases, sometimes CFS is erroneously diagnosed years later, as the connection between late-onset fatigue to the previous cancer diagnosis and treatment may not be immediately evident.

The Fatigue Coalition, an expert panel made up of medical practitioners, researchers, and patient advocates, has proposed formal diagnostic criteria for determining CrF and describing the symptoms, causes, and functional sequelae (Table 3.1) [1]. The proposed definition and diagnostic criteria were based on coalition members' clinical experience, survey results, and consensus-based discussion [1, 5]. First, fatigue must be prevalent for a period of at least 2 weeks during the preceding

**Table 3.1** Fatigue coalition diagnostic criteria for cancer-related fatigue

---

**A**: 2 weeks of significant fatigue in past month.

**B**: At least 5 of 10 of the following symptoms:

    1. General weakness or limb heaviness

    2. Diminished concentration or attention

    3. Decreased motivation or interest to engage in usual activities

    4. Insomnia or hypersomnia

    5. Non-restorative sleep

    6. Perceived need to struggle to overcome inactivity

    7. Marked emotional reactivity (e.g., sadness, frustration, or irritability) to feeling fatigued

    8. Difficulty completing daily tasks

    9. Perceived problems with short-term memory

    10. Post-exertional malaise

    The symptoms cause clinically significant distress or impairment in social, occupational, or other important areas of functioning.

**C**: Fatigue is a consequence of cancer or cancer therapy.

**D**: Fatigue is not a consequence of psychiatric comorbidity.

---

Criteria are based on International Classification of Diseases (ICD)-10 criteria [2]. (Adapted with permission from Cella et al. [1])

month, during which time significant fatigue or diminished energy was experienced each day (or almost every day), along with at least five (of ten) additional fatigue-related symptoms (Table 3.1). Second, the fatigue experienced results in significant distress or functional impairment. Third, there is clinical evidence suggesting fatigue is a consequence of cancer or cancer therapy. Fourth, fatigue is not primarily a consequence of a concurrent psychiatric condition (e.g., major depressive disorder) (Table 3.1) [1]. Donovan et al. systematically reviewed studies that reported results based on the use of the Fatigue Coalition diagnostic criteria and their findings validated and supported the reliability of the criteria [6].

## 3.3   Assessment Considerations

Due to the complex nature of CrF, a systematic assessment is essential for individual counseling and planning treatment strategies for each patient. Some specific characteristics of CrF may complicate the diagnostic process, such as [7]:

- non-specificity symptoms and signs of CrF, as they may also be due to other diseases or functional impairments;
- the patient's subjective feeling of his or her symptoms and impairments;
- patients with CrF often not appearing to be 'ill,' even if CrF has severe effects on their functional levels and health-related quality of life (HRQoL);
- the type and extent of symptoms varying markedly from one patient to another and changing over time; and
- lack of a validated laboratory test or biomarker to identify CrF.

Against this background, a comprehensive model of the etiology and pathogenesis as part of a multimodal assessment CrF is needed [7, 8]. This includes acceptance that several somatic and psychological factors may influence or contribute to CrF (Fig. 3.1) [9]. Thus, acknowledging the possibility of multiple contributing factors, the assessment approach should include clinical assessment (ie, presence of pain, anemia, insomnia, nutritional assessment, performance capacity, medications, comorbidities); psychological assessment (presence of depression, anxiety, emotional distress, coping mechanisms, non-cancer-related psychosocial distress); and self-rating (patients describing their personal circumstances via questionnaires).

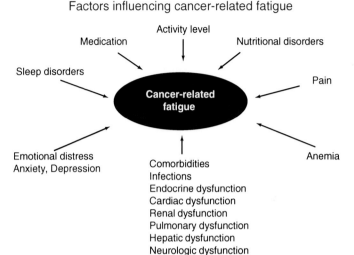

**Fig. 3.1** Assessment of factors influencing cancer-related fatigue. (Reproduced with permission from Mortimer et al. [9] © Journal of the National Comprehensive Cancer Network)

## 3.4 Clinical Assessment

Clinical assessment is at the center of the CrF diagnostic process. The physician should take a history of fatigue, including current status of disease, pretreatment activity levels, onset, pattern and duration, changes over time, and interference with function and activities of daily living. Additionally, the physician should consider contributing risk factors (e.g., mood disorders, pain, other comorbidities), carry out a physical examination, and review any fatigue symptoms with specific attention to a possible relationship to vegetative functions (e.g., sleep pattern, activity levels) and other factors such as social and environmental contributors; types of medication being taken; diet and nutrition; use of alcohol, tobacco, and recreational drugs; medical history before cancer (pre-existing fatigue); physical fitness; and sleep or other neurological disorders. It is also recommended to ask the patient whether the symptoms are new or unusual. Patient history, in combination with a physical examination, can provide important information and aid in identifying possible causes or contributing factors (Fig. 3.1) [10]. Although predictive values of laboratory tests are low in CrF, the following parameters should also be considered:

- serum electrolytes and glucose;
- transaminases and gamma-glutamyl transferase;
- C-reactive protein;
- red and white blood cell count/hemoglobin; and
- thyroid-stimulating hormone levels.

## 3.5   Psychological Assessment

Several studies have focused on correlation and comorbidity in CrF and psychiatric conditions, especially depression and anxiety [11–13]. As fatigue is a common symptom of both diagnostic efforts are required to reliably differentiate between CrF and these relatively common mood disorders [14–16]; for example, symptoms such as a loss of drive, sleeping disorders, and cognitive disorders overlap with secondary symptoms of depression. With respect to the course of CrF, it may be that chronic CrF can trigger a depressive episode. For instance, a continuing level of depression may be exacerbated by the distress of knowing that cancer is a life-threatening illness, as well as the stress of undergoing cancer treatment, which can cause both physical and emotional exhaustion. While the interactions between CrF and mood disorders have not yet been completely explained, a recent study on long-term fatigue discovered a possible psychological 'maladaption' to persisting effects of cancer and cancer treatment [17–19].

To date, only a few studies have investigated the complexity of interactions between physical and psychological aspects of CrF [16]. As such, physicians are often faced with the important task of determining a possible relationship between a patient with CrF and a psychiatric disorder such as depression. According to the findings of a study investigating breast cancer survivors, 6 months after completing cancer treatment, one-third of patients with CrF were also found to meet the criteria for major depression, as defined by the *Diagnostic and Statistical Manual of Mental Disorders* (DSM) [20]. As a consequence, it is thought that CrF can be both an expression of pre-existing depression and also a cause of depression. In clinical practice, a depressive disorder that underlies CrF can be detected rapidly and sensitively using two screening questions [21]:

- "In the last month, have you often felt dejected, sad, depressed, or hopeless?"
- "In the last month, have you derived much less pleasure than usual out of the things that you normally like to do?"

If the patient answers both questions affirmatively, a depressive disorder could be present and a further specialized psychiatric diagnostic evaluation is recommended.

## 3.6   Assessment Scales

Assessment of CrF is based on a comprehensive approach including clinical and psychological assessment, as well as the use of self-rating questionnaires and scales. It is recommended that cancer-specific fatigue scales are used instead of using generic fatigue scales. However, generic instruments may be used if the target of the assessment is to compare patients with cancer to those with other chronic diseases. While many of the fatigue scales have strengths and limitations, no clear recommendation can be made as to which measure is the most appropriate. Thus, although, there is no consensus 'gold standard' for measuring CrF, the self-report approach is the most common strategy in terms of assessment scales. Which instrument the clinician or researcher uses depends primarily on the setting and the goals of the assessment, with a multidimensional approach often favored. Overall, using a standardized questionnaire allows clinicians to measure CrF in the course over time and allows comparisons between various patient subgroups.

During the last decade, interest and research output in CrF has increased considerably and, therefore, more detailed instruments have been developed to assess CrF in patients with chronic diseases. In this overview, there will not be a focus on generic instrument developed for assessing fatigue in a non-cancer population, such as the Fatigue Feeling Checklist (FFB) [22] or Chalder Fatigue Scale [23]. Additionally, many cancer-specific instruments currently available are generic instruments and not recommended for CrF assessment. CrF-specific scales may be divided into two major subgroups: global instruments assessing overall health-related quality of life (HRQoL) and instruments specifically assessing CrF. Most of the global instruments assessing HRQoL include fatigue as single items or in sub-scales that specifically measure fatigue. These include:

- European Organization for Research and Treatment of Cancer Quality of Life Questionnaire, Version 3.0 (EORTC QLQ-C30): includes a one-dimensional fatigue subscale, including three fatigue items assessing the physical domain of fatigue [24];
- Profile of Mood States (POMS): has a 5-item fatigue subscale (multidimensional approach) measuring physical, emotional, and cognitive aspects of CrF [25];
- Breast Cancer Chemotherapy Questionnaire (BCQ): has a 3-item fatigue subscale [26];

- Cancer Rehabilitation Evaluation System (CARES): has a 3-item fatigue subscale [27];
- Short Form Health Survey (SF36): has a 4-item vitality subscale [28]; and
- Functional Assessment of Cancer Therapy: General (FACT-G): one fatigue-related item is measured (ie, lack of energy) [29].

Systematic reviews of specific questionnaires to assess CrF identified various scales and divided those instruments into unidimensional or multidimensional questionnaires [30, 31]. One-dimensional instruments such as the Functional Assessment of Chronic Illness Therapy – Fatigue (FACIT–F), a module developed by Cella et al. [5], or the Brief Fatigue Inventory (BFI), developed by Mendoza et al. [32], focus on physical symptoms of CrF, whereas multidimensional instruments such as the Multidimensional Fatigue Inventory [33] address the physical, emotional, and cognitive aspects of CrF. Most of the existing cancer-specific questionnaires are based on a multidimensional approach, which is in line with an understanding of CrF as a multifaceted syndrome [31].

While most of the scales pertain to intensity, some also measure interference with activities of daily living and/or HRQoL. However, sensitivity to change over time has been proven in only a few of these instruments [31, 33–35]. In general, there are a number of key psychometric criteria that need to be met in the assessment of fatigue to ensure meaningful results. However, not all existing fatigue measures fulfill these requirements and from 22 identified questionnaires that address CrF, only 14 have been validated to measure and meet a minimum quality score for inclusion as an assessment of fatigue [31].

The methodology used for developing the questionnaires often does not include any cross-cultural validation, despite the concept of fatigue differing from one country to another. Most of the instruments were developed in the United States with mainly Caucasian patients. However, in some cultures, the physical aspects of fatigue may be seen as more important than the social or psychological aspects. Thus, the existing questionnaires vary largely with respect to the criteria of validity, reliability, sensitivity to change, or cross-cultural applicability [30, 31]. Methods used for supporting claims of construct validity include known groups comparison and analyses for convergent and discriminant validity. Based on existing meta-analyses, a short overview of selected questionnaires for assessment of CrF will be given in this chapter.

### 3.6.1   Revised Piper Fatigue Scale

The Piper Fatigue Scale was initially developed in 1989 [36]. In 1998, as part of a larger study designed to measure subjective fatigue and influencing factors in women with breast cancer, Piper et al. decided to revise and reduce the scale via factor analysis [36]. The revised version of the Piper scale contains 22 items and refers to the patient's current situation, which is rated on an 11-point Likert scale. The Piper Scale includes four subscales: behavioral/severity, affective meaning, sensory, and cognitive/mood.

### 3.6.2   Fatigue Symptom Inventory

In 1998, Hann and colleagues developed and validated a self-report instrument for assessing both intensity and duration of fatigue in patients with cancer called the Fatigue Symptom Inventory (FSI) [34]. The FSI contains 13 items and covers four dimensions of fatigue: intensity, duration, daily pattern, and interference of fatigue. Patients answer each question on an 11-point rating scale.

### 3.6.3 Multidimensional Fatigue Inventory

Smets et al. developed the Multidimensional Fatigue Inventory (MFI) instrument in 1995 [33]. The MFI is a multidimensional 20-item self-report questionnaire. The authors postulated five dimensions of fatigue based on the manner in which fatigue may be expressed: general fatigue, physical fatigue, mental fatigue, reduced motivation, and reduced activity, with an equal number of questions for each dimension [37]. Patients used a 7-point Likert Scale to rate the extent to which a particular question applied ('*yes, that is true*' to '*no, that is not true*'). The scale has demonstrated good internal consistency ($\alpha = 0.8$) and a high construct validity, and was assessed in an initial validation study using disease-free patients that had finished radiation therapy for cancer [38].

An expanded inventory, the Multidimensional Fatigue Symptom Inventory (MFSI), was developed in 2001 and includes five symptom dimensions of fatigue including global experience, somatic symptoms, cognitive symptoms, affective symptoms, and behavioral symptoms [39]. The expanded MFSI consists of 83 items and takes approximately 5–10 min to complete, with respondents rating each statement for the past 7 days on a 5-point scale (0 = not at all; 4 = extremely).

### 3.6.4 Brief Fatigue Inventory

The BFI is a 9-item questionnaire developed by Mendoza and colleagues for rapid assessment of fatigue severity for use in both clinical screening and clinical trials [32] (Fig. 3.2). The BFI was developing using data collected by the Pain Research Group at the Wisconsin Comprehensive Cancer Center and a review of the literature. The nine items are measured on an 11-point scale (0 = no fatigue; 10 = as bad as you can imagine). The BFI was shown to be a reliable measure for assessing the severity of fatigue [32].

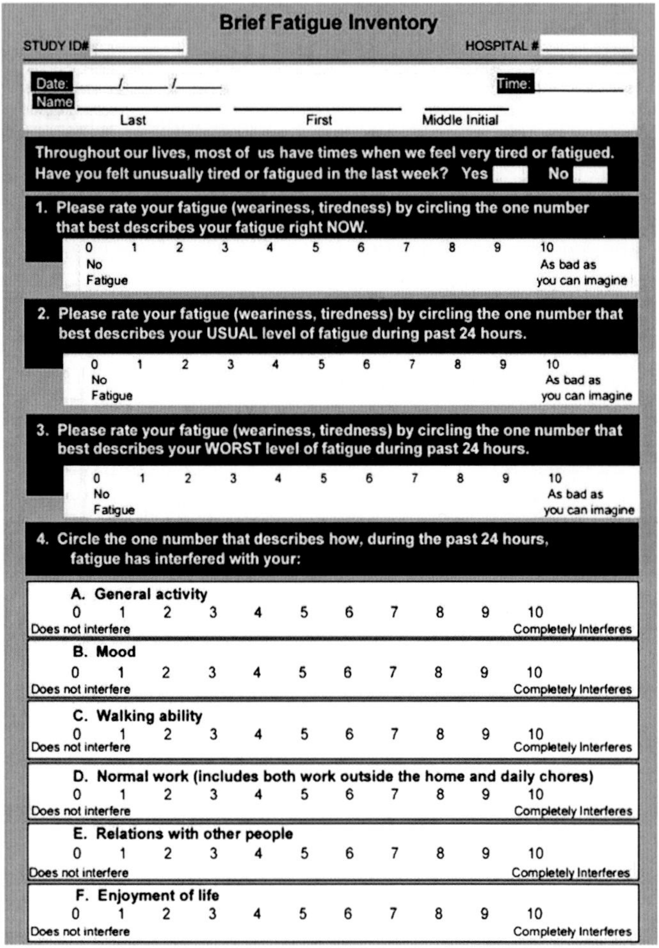

**Fig. 3.2** Brief Fatigue Inventory. (Reproduced with permission from Mendoza et al. [32]©John Wiley and Sons)

### 3.6.5   Schwartz Cancer Fatigue Scale

In 1998, Anna Schwartz developed a multidimensional measure of CrF that incorporated Piper's Integrated Fatigue Model and Crimprich's Attentional Fatigue Theory to form the Schwartz Cancer Fatigue Scale [35]. It is a questionnaire that consists of 28 self-rated items with a 5-point Likert scale that ranges from 'not at all' to 'extremely.' The following key dimensions were identified by an initial factor analysis: physical (e.g., neurophysiological aspects), emotional (e.g., loss of ability, feeling of helplessness, and vulnerability), cognitive (e.g., ability to direct attention) and temporal (e.g., classification of acute and chronic fatigue) [40, 41].

### 3.6.6   Functional Assessment of Cancer Therapy – Fatigue Scale

The Functional Assessment of Cancer Therapy-Fatigue (FACT-F) instrument was developed by David Cella in 1997. The FACT-F is composed of a core questionnaire (Functional Assessment of Cancer Therapy - General) plus a subscale with 13 fatigue-specific items. The core questionnaire was developed by Cella and colleagues [29] and a number of adapted versions are available. The FACT-F contains items assessing weakness, listlessness, need for sleep, and tiredness that imposes limits on activity. The scale has high reliable internal consistency ($r = .95$), making the fatigue subscale suitable for individual use [42].

### 3.6.7   Fatigue Assessment Questionnaire

The Fatigue Assessment Questionnaire was developed in 1998 to measure the nature of fatigue in patients with cancer [43].

This instrument contains 20 items distributed among 3 dimensions: physical, emotional, and cognitive. Patients detail their fatigue status during the past week on a 4-point Likert scale and across three visual analog scales.

### 3.6.8 Cancer Fatigue Scale

The Cancer Fatigue Scale (CFS) was developed in 2000 by Okuyama and colleagues in Japan [44]. It consists of 15 items which are answered on a 5-point Likert scale with regard to the patient's experiences during the past week. The three subscales (physical, affective, and cognitive) have been shown to be valid and the mean value of the correlation coefficient between the CFS and a visual analog scale for fatigue was 0.67 ($P < 0.001$) [44].

### 3.6.9 European Organization for Research and Treatment of Cancer Quality of Life Questionnaire – Fatigue

Within the last decade, the European Organization for Research and Treatment of Cancer Quality of Life Questionnaire – Fatigue (EORTC QLQ Fa13) questionnaire, an additional scale for assessment of CrF, was developed to be used in conjunction with the EORTC core questionnaire used to measure quality of life in patients with cancer (EORTC QLQ 30) [45, 46]. It is a multidimensional instrument including 13 items; 2 items are global items, whereas 11 measure impact of CrF on physical, emotional, and cognitive levels in accordance with the EORTC guidelines. A summary of the assessment scales used in cancer-related fatigue can be found in Table 3.2.

**Table 3.2** Assessment scales used for cancer-related fatigue

| Name of the scale [reference] | Measures for: | Dimension(s) | Number of items |
|---|---|---|---|
| Piper Fatigue Scale (PFS) [36, 47] | Intensity, interference with activities of daily living | Multidimensional (time, sensory, affective) | 20 (revised form) |
| Multidimensional Fatigue Inventory (MFI) [37] | Intensity | Multidimensional approach: general fatigue, physical, mental, reduced activity, reduced motivation | 20 |
| Functional Assessment of Cancer Therapy – Fatigue scale (FACT-F) [5] | Intensity | One dimension: physical | 7 |
| Fatigue Symptom Inventory (FSI) [34] | Intensity, duration and interference with activities of daily living (ADL). | Multidimensional structure | 13 |
| Brief Fatigue Inventory (BFI) [32] | Intensity, interference with ADL | One dimension | 9 |
| Schwartz Cancer Fatigue Scale (SCFS) [35] | Intensity | Multidimensional: physical, emotional, cognitive, | 28 (short form 6) |
| Fatigue Assessment Questionnaire (FAQ) [43] | Intensity | Multidimensional: physical, affective, cognitive | 20 |
| Cancer Fatigue Scale (CFS) [44] | Intensity | Multidimensional: physical, affective, cognitive | 15 |
| EORTC QLQ Fa13 Module [45] | Intensity, interference | Multidimensional: physical, emotional, cognitive | 13 |

## 3.7   Assessment Procedures

According to current guidelines, patients with cancer should be asked directly about fatigue symptoms at regular intervals during treatment and follow-up and assessed using a self-rating scale [8, 48]. As a first step, the use of a linear analog scale is recommended for recording the intensity of symptoms (e.g., $0 =$ no fatigue; $10 =$ worst fatigue you can imagine). For most scales, a reported intensity of $\geq 4$ is taken as the threshold value for further diagnostic assessment [49, 50]. Depending on the screening score, further assessment using one of the questionnaires described above could be helpful for identifying CrF, as well as determining the severity of the symptoms.

## References

1. Cella D, Davis K, Breitbart W, Curt G. Cancer-related fatigue: prevalence of proposed diagnostic criteria in a United States Sample of cancer survivors. J Clin Oncol. 2001;19:3385–91.
2. World Health Organization (WHO). International Classification of Diseases (ICD-10). 2013. WHO website. www.who.int/classifications/icd10/browse/2010/en. Accessed 25 September 2014.
3. Yancey JR, Thomas SM. Chronic fatigue syndrome: diagnosis and treatment. Am Fam Physician. 2012;86:741–6.
4. Moss-Morris R, Deary V, Castell B. Chronic fatigue syndrome. Handb Clin Neurol. 2013;110:303–14.
5. Cella D. The functional assessment of Cancer Therapy Anemia and Fatigue Scale: a new tool for the assessment of outcomes in cancer anemia and fatigue. Semin Hematol. 1997;34:13–9.
6. Donovan K, McGinty H, Jacobsen P. A systematic review of research using diagnostic criteria for cancer-related fatigue. Psychooncology. 2013;22:737–44.
7. Horneber M, Fischer I, Dimeo F, Rüffer JU, Weis J. Cancer-related fatigue epidemiology, pathogenesis, diagnosis, and treatment. Dtsch Arztebl Int. 2012;109:161–72.

8. National Comprehensive Cancer Network (NCCN). Clinical practice guidelines in oncology: cancer related fatigue. Version 1. 2014. www.nccn.org/professionals/physician_gls/f_guidelines.asp. Accessed 25 September 2014.

9. Mortimer JE, Barsevick AM, Bennett CL, et al. Studying cancer-related fatigue: report of the NCCN Scientific Research Committee. J Natl Compr Canc Netw. 2010;8:1331–9.

10. Bruera E. Cancer-related fatigue: a multidimensional syndrome. J Support Oncol. 2010;8:175–6.

11. Patrick DL, Ferketich SL, Frame PS, et al. National Institutes of Health state-of-the-science conference statement: symptom management in cancer: pain, depression, and fatigue, July 15–17, 2002. J Natl Cancer Inst. 2003;95:1110–7.

12. Valentine A, Meyers C. Cognitive and mood disturbance as causes and symptoms of fatigue in cancer patients. Cancer. 2001;96 suppl 6:1694–8.

13. Visser M, Smets E. Fatigue, depression and quality of life in cancer patients: how are they related? Support Care Cancer. 1998;6:101–8.

14. Hayes J. Depression and chronic fatigue in cancer patients. Prim Care. 1991;18:327–39.

15. Gaston-Johansson F, Fall-Dickson J, Bakos A, Kennedy M. Fatigue, pain, and depression in pre-autotransplant breast cancer patients. Cancer Pract. 1999;7:240–7.

16. Brown LF, Kroenke K. Cancer-related fatigue and its associations with depression and anxiety: a systematic review. Psychosomatics. 2009;50:440–7.

17. Rich TA. Symptom clusters in cancer patients and their relation to EGFR ligand modulation of the circadian axis. J Support Oncol. 2007;5:167–74.

18. Ancoli-Israel S, Moore PJ, Jones V. The relationship between fatigue and sleep in cancer patients: a review. Eur J Cancer Care. 2001;10:245–55.

19. Wettergren L, Langius A, Björkholm M, Björvell H. Physical and psychosocial functioning in patients undergoing autologous bone marrow transplantation – a prospective study. Bone Marrow Transplant. 1997;20:497–502.

20. Andrykowski MA, Donovan KA, Laronga C, Jacobsen PB. Prevalence, predictors, and characteristics of off-treatment fatigue in breast cancer survivors. Cancer. 2010;116:5740–8.

21. Whooley MA, Avins AL, Miranda J, Browner WS. Case finding instruments for depression: two questions are as good as many. J Gen Intern Med. 1997;12:439–45.

22. Pearson RG, Byars GE. The development and validation of a checklist measuring subjective fatigue. Air University, School of Aviation Medicine, US Air Force, Randolph Air Force Base, Texas, Document No. 56115;1956.

23. Chalder T, Berelowitz G, Pawlikowska T, et al. Development of a fatigue scale. J Psychosom Res. 1993;37:147–53.

24. Aaronson NK, Ahmedzai S, Bergman B, et al. The European Organization for Research and Treatment of Cancer QLQ-C30: a quality-of-life instrument for use in international clinical trials in oncology. J Natl Cancer Inst. 1993;85:365–76.

25. McNair DM, Lorr M, Dropplemann LF. The manual for the profile of mood states. San Diego, CA: Educational and Industrial Testing Service; 1971.

26. Levine MN, Guyatt GH, Gent M, et al. Quality of life in stage II breast cancer: an instrument for clinical trials. J Clin Oncol. 1988;6:1798–810.

27. Schag CAC, Heinrich RL. Cancer Rehabilitation Evaluation System (CARES) manual. Los Angeles: CARES Consultants; 1988.

28. Ware Jr JE, Sherbourne CD. The MOS 36-item short-form health survey (SF-36). I. Conceptual framework and item selection. Med Care. 1992;30:473–83.

29. Cella DF, Tulsky DS, Gray G, et al. The Functional Assessment of Cancer Therapy scale: development and validation of the general measure. J Clin Oncol. 1993;11:570–9.

30. Ahlberg K, Ekman T, Gaston-Johansson F, Mock V. Assessment and management of cancer-related fatigue in adults. Lancet. 2003;362:640–50.

31. Minton O, Stone P. A systematic review of the scales used for the measurement of cancer-related fatigue (CRF). Ann Oncol. 2009;20:17–25.

32. Mendoza TR, Wang XS, Kugaya A, et al. The rapid assessment of fatigue severity in cancer patients; use of the brief Fatigue Inventory. Cancer. 1999;85:1186–96.

33. Smets EMA, Garssen B, Bonke B, De Haes JCJM. The Multidimensional Fatigue Inventory (MFI) psychometric qualities of an instrument to assess fatigue. J Psychom Res. 1995;39:315–25.

34. Hann DM, Jacobsen PB, Azzarello LM, et al. Measurement of fatigue in cancer patients: development and validation of the Fatigue Symptom Inventory. Qual Life Res. 1998;7:301–10.

35. Schwartz JE, Jandorf L, Krupp LB. The measurement of fatigue: a new instrument. J Psychosom Res. 1993;37:753–62.

36. Piper BF, Dibble SL, Dodd MJ, Weiss MC, Slaughter RE, Paul SM. The revised Piper Fatigue Scale: psychometric evaluation in women with breast cancer. Oncol Nurs Forum. 1998;25:677–84.

37. Smets EMA, Visser MRM, Willems-Groot AFMN, et al. Fatigue and radiotherapy: experience in patients undergoing treatment. Br J Cancer. 1998;78:899–906.

38. Smets EMA, Visser MRM, Willems-Groot AFMN, Garssen B, Schuster-Uitterhoeve ALJ, de Haes JCJM. Fatigue and radiotherapy: experience in patients 9 months following treatment. Br J Cancer. 1998;78:907–12.

39. Stein KD, Martin SC, Hann DM, Jacobsen PB. A multidimensional measure of fatigue for use with cancer patients. Cancer Pract. 1998;6: 143–52.

40. Schwartz AL. The Schwartz Cancer Fatigue Scale. Testing reliability and validity. Oncol Nurs Forum. 1998;25:711–7.

41. Schwartz AL, Meek PM, Nail LM. Measurement of fatigue: determining minimal important differences. J Clin Epidemiol. 2002;55:239–44.

42. Yellen SB, Cella DF, Webster K, Blendowski C, Kaplan E. Measuring fatigue and other anemia-related symptoms with the Functional Assessment of Cancer Therapy (FACT) measurement system. J Pain Symptom Manage. 1997;13:63–74.

43. Glaus A. Fatigue in patients with cancer: analysis and assessment. Recent results Cancer Res. Heidelberg: Springer; 1998.

44. Okuyama T, Akechi T, Kugaya A, et al. Development and validation of the Cancer Fatigue Scale: a brief, three-dimensional, self-rating scale for assessment of fatigue in cancer patients. J Pain Symptom Manage. 2000;19:5–14.

45. Weis J, Arraras JI, Conroy T, et al. Development of an EORTC quality of life phase III module measuring cancer-related fatigue (EORTC QLQ-FA13). Psychooncology. 2013;22:1002–7.

46. European Organization for Research and Treatment of Cancer (EORTC). 2013. EORTC Quality of Life Questionnaire. Version 30. EORTC website. http://groups.eortc.be/qol/eortc-qlq-c30. Accessed 25 September 2014.

47. Piper BF, Lindsey AM, Dodd MJ, Ferketich S, Paul SM, Weller S. The development of an instrument to measure the subjective dimension of fatigue. In: Funk SG, Tournquist EM, Champagne MT, Copp LA, Weise RA, editors. Key aspects of comfort: management of pain, fatigue, and nausea. New York: Springer; 1989. p. 199–208.

48. Howell D, Keller-Olaman S, Oliver TK, et al. A pan-Canadian practice guideline and algorithm: screening, assessment, and supportive care of adults with cancer-related fatigue. Curr Oncol. 2013;20:e233–46

49. Given B, Given CW, Sikorskii A, et al. Establishing mild, moderate, and severe scores for cancer-related symptoms: how consistent and clinically meaningful are interference-based severity cutpoints? J Pain Symptom Manage. 2008;35:126–35.

50. Butt Z, Wagner LI, Beaumont JL. Use of a single item screening instrument to detect clinically relevant fatigue, distress, pain and anorexia in ambulatory cancer practice. J Pain Symptom Manage. 2008;35:20–30.

# Chapter 4
# Nonpharmacological Treatment

## 4.1 Introduction

A growing body of scientific evidence supports the use of non-pharmacological treatment strategies for alleviating cancer-related fatigue (CrF) [1, 2]. Nonpharmacological treatments include a variety of interventions such as psychosocial support, stress management, energy conservation, nutritional therapy, sleep therapy, and exercise. These interventions comprise a variety of multimodal interventions and can be summarized into three major categories:

- psychosocial interventions;
- mind-body interventions; and
- exercise and sports therapy.

## 4.2 Psychosocial Interventions

Psychosocial interventions for treating CrF cover a broad range of interventions such as psychosocial counseling, psychotherapy, or psycho-education. Apart from communicating information

J. Weis, M. Horneber, *Cancer-Related Fatigue*,
DOI 10.1007/978-1-907673-76-4_4,
© Springer Healthcare 2015

about CrF, the main goals of those interventions are to help patients restructure their cognitive appraisal of CrF, change their coping strategies and behavior, and address self-help or self-care strategies. Some of those interventions include elements such as relaxation techniques, energy conservation, and stress management. Most of the psychosocial interventions may be carried out as both individual and group interventions.

## *4.2.1   Information and Counseling*

Information and counseling can help patients obtain a better understanding of CrF, not only as a possible result of cancer and treatment, but also as a condition influenced by various other factors. As a first step, information on the multifactorial nature of CrF, and its potential causes and influencing factors, should be given. Once armed with this information, counseling from a physician can also help patients to devise a personalized activity plan, taking restrictions due to CrF into account. Counseling should include recommendations for energy preservation, task prioritization, activity pacing, and advice on how to delegate less important activities [3, 4]. There is some evidence that such strategies can improve quality of life and reduce the subjective feeling of fatigue [4]. Information and counseling may be supported by brochures or interactive media, including internet platforms which are often provided by national cancer societies. It is also recommended to inform and educate patients with cancer about ways to prevent fatigue or avoid it becoming a chronic condition [5]. Information and counseling should be provided not only for the individual patient but also for partners or family members, which can help prevent negative psychosocial implications, such as misunderstandings and emotional withdrawal.

**Table 4.1** Psychoeducational interventions for cancer-related fatigue

| |
| --- |
| Identify and diminish sources of psychosocial distress |
| Differentiate between symptoms of fatigue and depression |
| Identify patterns associated with fatigue |
| Set aside periods of rest and activity during the day |
| Schedule important daily activities to maximize efficiency |
| Identify and minimize fatigue-exacerbating activities |
| Devise an activity/exercise program |
| Practice good sleep hygiene |
| Set realistic activity goals |
| Partake in self-restoring activities and identify potential resources |
| Maintain communication with partners, family members, and social network (including sharing feelings of fatigue) |

### *4.2.2 Psychoeducation*

Psychoeducational interventions should focus on the management of CrF and help patients to promote self-management, adaptation, and adjustment to their current condition and any treatment sequelae [6]. The most important goal of psychoeducational intervention is to facilitate self-care for the person with cancer [7]. Recognizing that emotional distress is highly correlated with fatigue, psychoeducational interventions should focus on identification of coping strategies to optimize a patient's ability to deal with anxiety, depression, and psychosocial distress. Specific techniques for the management of fatigue are presented in Table 4.1 [8–10].

It is often helpful for patients to identify sources of psychosocial distress and to eliminate stress-producing activities where possible. Additionally, because there can be symptom overlap between CrF and depression, the patient should be supported to differentiate between the two often similar conditions. Sleep disorders are a common result of cancer-related distress and can be a contributing factor to CrF. Thus, patients should be also encouraged to observe sleeping behavior and practice good sleep hygiene. This includes avoiding lying in bed other than to sleep, going to bed and rising at the same time each day, and avoiding stimulants that can disrupt sleep.

Another important element is for patients to recognize patterns of fatigue and find a balance between rest and activity during the day. This can be done by using diary techniques, including subjective rating of each activity in terms of the perceived level of fatigue that follows. These techniques can help a patient identify fatigue-promoting activities and develop specific strategies to avoid or modify them. Patients should be encouraged to schedule important daily activities according to the period of lowest experienced fatigue over the day which involves setting priorities and maintaining a reasonable schedule. Health professionals may also assist patients by providing information on support services that are available to help with daily activities and responsibilities.

Patients should be supported in partaking in self-restoring activities and setting realistic goals to avoid frustration. For example, an important part of patient psychoeducation should be encouraging regular exercise and explaining the benefits, while still recognizing individual limitations and their level of physical fitness. This can be included in the development of an individual activity/rest program based on an assessment of the patient's fatigue patterns that allows the best use of the individual's energy. A good example is relaxation techniques and meditation, which may even target underlying biologic mechanisms and reduce cancer-related distress by diminishing activation of the hypothalamic-pituitary-adrenal (HPA) axis [11, 12]. Another example is yoga, which will be discussed later in this chapter.

Outcomes of psychoeducational programs have been investigated in several studies [13]. In a controlled trial of patients with pain and fatigue during chemotherapy, a behavioral intervention in which nurses engaged patients with problem-solving approaches to symptom management aimed at improving physical functioning and emotional health, lead to marked improvements in quality of life and decreased symptom burden when compared with standard care [14]. A meta-analysis of 119 trials by Kangas et al. demonstrated that many counseling and educational interventions were found to substantially improve vigor/vitality and reduce fatigue, although often only with a small-to-moderate effect on overall CrF (which was often a secondary endpoint) [15]. Additionally, in Goedentorp et al., five CrF-specific intervention studies which consisted of psychoeducational elements such as education about fatigue, teaching self-care or coping techniques, and activity management were analyzed; in most of those studies, the authors demonstrated a measurable reduction in CrF [16].

### 4.2.3 Cognitive Behavioral Therapy

Cognitive behavioral therapy (CBT) is an intervention that addresses emotions, behaviors, and cognitive processes, and applies them toward goal-oriented and systematic activities. CBT in CrF takes into account the thoughts and functional behaviors relevant to the syndrome and focuses on the individual and their pattern of psychological factors [17]. CBT is generally used post-treatment, but may be also used for patients with CrF still undergoing chemotherapy [18]. Based on existing literature and experience in clinical practice, CBT is generally used to address the following factors:

- coping with the experience of cancer [19];
- fear of disease recurrence [10, 20];
- dysfunctional thoughts and beliefs regarding fatigue [21, 22];
- sleep dysregulation [23, 24];
- activity dysregulation [10, 20, 24]; and
- low level of social support/negative social interactions [22].

There have been several studies to evaluate CBT, but fatigue has only been investigated as primary outcome in a handful of them [14, 18, 25]. In those studies, the number of therapy sessions varied according to the number of focused topics (range: 5–26 1-hour sessions; mean: 12.5 sessions) and showed a clinically significant decrease in fatigue severity and functional impairment. For example, Kangas et al. showed that among psychosocial randomized controlled trials that reported fatigue or vigor/vitality as outcome criteria, approximately 40 % of the studies using CBT interventions were found to significantly increase vigor/vitality and two-thirds significantly reduced fatigue [15]. In addition, it has been have demonstrated that among psychosocial treatment approaches, cognitive-behavioral interventions are the most effective against CrF [16, 17]. In summary, CBT may be regarded as a useful strategy, especially for persisting CrF.

## 4.3   Mind-Body Interventions

### 4.3.1   Mindfulness-Based Stress Reduction

Mindfulness-based clinical interventions are mind-body modalities that combine meditation exercises with psycho-educational elements, cognitive-behavioral interventions, and movement exercises [26]. The core practices are sitting meditation with breath awareness and focused attention, awareness of sensations in the body (body scan), yoga exercises (e.g., hatha yoga, mindful movement), walking meditation, and insight meditation. The two most commonly used mindfulness-based clinical interventions in oncology are mindfulness-based stress reduction (MBSR) and mindfulness-based cognitive therapy (MBCT).

MBSR is a specific multimodal program focused on improving well-being and health [26]. Based on the eastern meditation practice of Zen Buddhism, the MBSR program was developed by Professor Kabat-Zinn at the Massachusetts Medical Center [26]. The program includes one 90-minute session per week for 8 weeks, along with a 3-hour 'silent retreat' between week 6 and week 7. A recent meta-analysis on the effects of MBSR on mental and physical health status of patients with cancer showed positive outcomes for mental health (Cohen's $d$ effect size = 0.48) [27]. Documented benefits included improvements in stress, mood, anxiety, sleep, fatigue, psychological functioning, psychosocial adjustment, coping, well-being, quality of life, and fear of recurrence after program participation [28–30]. Most of the studies did not specifically use CrF reduction as an trial endpoint, but it was included as part of a combination of multiple health-related. However, recent studies have shown that MBSR may indeed be helpful for improving CrF [31–33].

## 4.3.2  Yoga

Yoga is a mind-body intervention comprised of a combination of physical poses with a focus on breathing and meditation [34]. It is thought to have beneficial effects on physical and emotional health and has been used as an intervention to reduce CrF. There are several studies in which the benefits of yoga have been investigated in patients with cancer, with most addressing multimodal outcome criteria, including fatigue [35–37]. In a meta-analysis by Lin et al., 4 of the 10 studies included in the review used fatigue as an outcome measure but overall improvement of fatigue of the yoga-practicing groups was not found to be significant ($P=0.24$) [34]. In contrast, Buffart et al. [38] found yoga had a moderate-to-significant effect size on fatigue ($d=-0.51$). This is in line with Bower et al. which found beneficial effects – decline in fatigue severity, increased vigor – on persistent fatigue in breast cancer survivors after 12 weeks of yoga classes when compared to controls [39]. Although patients practicing yoga may perceive improvements in quality of life, fatigue, stress, anxiety, and depression, there needs to be additional randomized-controlled studies, especially with outcome criteria specific to CrF [38].

## 4.4    Exercise and Sports Therapy

Almost counter-intuitively, exercise has been shown to be an effective treatment strategy for CrF. However, patients diagnosed with cancer often become physically less active, which may increase fatigue [40, 41]. This is because when patients become less physically active, they are more easily fatigued, and when patients experience fatigue, they often react by becoming even less physically active. This negative spiral can be interrupted by improving the physical activity of the patients [42]. Interventions to promote and reinforce activity, exercise, and physical training have been proven to be effective against the continuing decrease of physical functional status [43–46]. Within the last decade, several reviews and meta-analyses have demonstrated substantial evidence that moderate training, often in combination with relaxation techniques and body awareness, can help reduce subjective fatigue levels. A systematic review showed moderate effects of physical training especially for some patient subgroups if applied during and after cancer treatment [44]. Physical activity frequency and intensity should be carried out in an individualized fashion depending on the patient's age, clinical status of cancer, and level of fitness [42].

Exercise programs should include elements of strength and endurance training to help the patient escape from the 'vicious circle' of physical inactivity, deconditioning, and rapid

**Table 4.2** Contraindications of exercise programs for patients with cancer-related fatigue

| |
|---|
| **Absolute contraindications (do not exercise)** |
|   Acute illnesses |
|   Acute worsening or decompensation of a chronic illness |
|   Fever above 38°C |
|   Acute pain |
|   Inadequately controlled arterial hypertension |
| **Relative contraindications (use caution)** |
|   Anemia (hemoglobin below 8 g/dL) |
|   Thrombocytopenia, coagulopathy |
|   Bone metastases |
|   Chronic illnesses such as coronary heart disease, occlusive peripheral arterial disease, arterial hypertension, diabetes mellitus, arthrosis |
|   Administration of cytostatic agents on the same day |
|   Mediastinal/cardiac radiation therapy |
|   Flu-like symptoms under immunotherapy |
|   Epilepsy |

exhaustion. National Comprehensive Cancer Network (NCCN) [47] guidelines recommend physical exercise sessions several times per week, along with daily endurance exercises and twice-weekly strength exercises. Each training session should last 30–45 minutes, according to the physical limitations of the individual and involve exercises that elevate heart rate to 70–80 % of maximum capacity. Patients with CrF should consider all relevant contraindications before starting an exercise regime [42] (Table 4.2).

It is useful to encourage patients to practice their favorite types of physical exercise and to adapt the intensity and duration of each training session to their current physical situation. Apart from physical limitations, additional patient barriers to physical activity include a lack of interest and motivation, as well as a purported lack of opportunity [48]. The health professional should detect any potential barriers and facilitate opportunities for the patient, including the use of CBT techniques in combination with or to encourage exercise [19]. The main objective is to help the patient to make physical exercise a regular part of their daily routine, keeping in mind that exercise-based interventions should be multidimensional and individualized according to health outcome and cancer type [45].

After diagnosis (see Chap. 3), appropriate interventions for the patient must be decided, with consideration of patient clinical status. Patients with cancer currently under treatment or immediately after treatment may benefit more from information and counseling, whereas patients in rehabilitation or long-term survivors may profit from combined CBT and exercise programs, for example. Patients with progressive, terminal disease may benefit most from pharmacological treatment, combined with information and counseling. There remains a need for well-designed, specific intervention studies to evaluate the direct effects of nonpharmacological interventions aimed at decreasing CrF.

# References

1. Mustian K, Morrow G, Carroll J, Figueroa-Moseley C, Jean-Pierre P, Williamse G. Integrative nonpharmacologic behavioral interventions for the management of cancer-related fatigue. Oncologist. 2007;12: 52–67.
2. Mitchell SA, Beck SL, Hood LE, et al. Putting evidence into practise: evidence-based interventions for fatigue during and following cancer and its treatment. Clin J Oncol Nurs. 2007;11:99–113.
3. Hinds PS, Quargneti A, Bush AJ, et al. An evaluation of the impact of a self-care coping intervention on psychological and clinical outcomes in adolescents with newly diagnosed cancer. Eur J Oncol Nurs. 2000; 4:6–19.
4. Barsevick AM, Dudley W, Beck S, et al. A randomized clinical trial of energy conservation for patients with cancer-related fatigue. Cancer. 2004;100:1302–10.
5. Godino C, Jodar L, Duran A, Martinez I, Schiaffino A. Nursing education as an intervention to decrease fatigue perception in oncology patients. Eur J Oncol Nurs. 2006;10:150–5.

6. Boesen EH, Ross L, Frederiksen K, et al. Psychoeducational intervention for patients with cutaneous malignant melanoma: a replication study. J Clin Oncol. 2005;23:1270–7.

7. Williams SA, Schreier AM. The role of education in managing fatigue, anxiety, and sleep disorders in women undergoing chemotherapy for breast cancer. Appl Nurs Res. 2005;18:138–47.

8. Yuen HK, Mitcham M, Morgan L. Managing post-therapy fatigue for cancer survivors using energy conservation training. J Allied Health. 2006;35:E121–39.

9. Ream E, Richardson A, Alexander-Dann C. Supportive intervention for fatigue in patients undergoing chemotherapy: a randomized controlled trial. J Pain Symptom Manage. 2006;31:148–61.

10. Yates P, Aranda S, Hargraves M, et al. Randomized controlled trial of an educational intervention for managing fatigue in women receiving adjuvant chemotherapy for early-stage breast cancer. J Clin Oncol. 2005;23:6027–36.

11. Stanton AL, Ganz PA, Kwan L, et al. Outcomes from the moving beyond cancer psychoeducational, randomized, controlled trial with breast cancer patients. J Clin Oncol. 2005;23:6009–18.

12. Kim SD, Kim HS. Effects of a relaxation breathing exercise on fatigue in haemopoietic stem cell transplantation patients. J Clin Nurs. 2005; 14:51–5.

13. Jacobsen PB, Donovan KA, Vadaparamil ST, Small BJ. Systematic review and meta-analysis of psychological and activity-based interventions for cancer-related fatigue. Health Psychol. 2007;26:660–7.

14. Given B, Given CW, McCorkle R, et al. Pain and fatigue management: results of a nursing randomized clinical trial. Oncol Nurs Forum. 2002; 29:949–56.

15. Kangas M, Bovbjerg DH, Montgomery GH. Cancer-related fatigue: a systematic and meta-analytic review of nonpharmacological therapies for cancer patients. Psychol Bull. 2008;134:700–41.

16. Goedendorp MM, Gielissen MF, Verhagen CA, Bleijenberg G. Psychosocial interventions for reducing fatigue during cancer treatment in adults. Cochrane Database Syst Rev. 2009:CD006953.

17. Gielissen MFM, Verhagen S, Witjes AJ, Bleijenberg G. The effects of cognitive behavior therapy in severely fatigued disease-free cancer patients compared to patients waiting for this treatment. A randomized controlled trial. J Clin Oncol. 2006;24:4882–7.

18. Given C, Given B, Rahbar M, et al. Effect of a cognitive behavioral intervention on reducing symptom severity during chemotherapy. J Clin Oncol. 2004;22:507–16.

19. Gielissen MF, Schattenberg AV, Verhagen CA, Rinkes MJ, Bremmers ME, Bleijenberg G. Experience of severe fatigue in long-term survivors

of stem cell transplantation. Bone Marrow Transplant. 2007;39: 595–603.

20. Servaes P, Verhagen C, Bleijenberg G. Fatigue in cancer patients during and after treatment: prevalence, correlates and interventions. Eur J Cancer. 2002;38:27–43.

21. Broeckel JA, Jacobsen PB, Horton J, Balducci L, Lyman GH. Characteristics and correlates of fatigue after adjuvant chemotherapy for breast cancer. J Clin Oncol. 1998;16:1689–96.

22. Servaes P, Verhagen C, Bleijenberg G. Determinants of chronic fatigue in disease-free breast cancer patients: a cross-sectional study. Ann Oncol. 2002;13:589–98.

23. Servaes P, Prins J, Verhagen S, Bleijenberg G. Fatigue after breast cancer and in chronic fatigue syndrome: similarities and differences. J Psychosom Res. 2002;52:453–9.

24. Prue G, Rankin J, Allen J, Gracey J, Cramp F. Cancer related fatigue: a critical appraisal. Eur J Cancer. 2006;42:846–63.

25. Given BA, Given CW, Jeon S, et al. Effect of neutropenia on the impact of a cognitive-behavioral intervention for symptom management. Cancer. 2005;104:869–78.

26. Kabat-Zinn J. An outpatient program in behavioral medicine for chronic pain patients based on the practice of mindfulness meditation: theoretical considerations and preliminary results. Gen Hosp Psychiatry. 1982;4:33–47.

27. Ledesma D, Kumano H. Mindfulness-based stress reduction and cancer: a meta-analysis. Psychooncology. 2009;18:571–9.

28. Shennan C, Payne S, Fenlon D. What is the evidence for the use of mindfulness-based interventions in cancer care? A review. Psychooncology. 2011;20:681–97.

29. Speca M, Carlson LE, Goodey E, et al. A randomized wait-list controlled clinical trial: the effect of a mindfulness meditation-based stress reduction program on mood and symptoms of stress in cancer outpatients. Psychosom Med. 2000;62:613–22.

30. Carlson LE, Speca M, Patel KD, et al. Mindfulness-based stress reduction in relation to quality of life, mood, symptoms of stress and levels of cortisol, dehydroepiandrosterone sulfate (DHEAS) and melatonin in breast and prostate cancer outpatients. Psychoneuroendocrinology. 2004;29:448–74.

31. Carlson LE, Garland SN. Impact of mindfulness-based stress reduction (MBSR) on sleep, mood, stress and fatigue symptoms in cancer outpatients. Int J Behav Med. 2005;12:278–85.

32. Lengacher CA, Johnson-Mallard V, Post-White J, Moscoso MS, Jacobsen PB, Klein TW, et al. Randomized controlled trial of

mindfulness-based stress reduction (MBSR) for survivors of breast cancer. Psychooncology. 2009;18:1261–72.

33. Lengacher CA, Reich RR, Post-White J, Moscoso M, Shelton MM, Barta M, et al. Mindfulness based stress reduction in post-treatment breast cancer patients: an examination of symptoms and symptom clusters. J Behav Med. 2012;35:86–94.

34. Lin KY, Hu YT, Chang KJ, Lin HF, Tsauo JY. Effects of yoga on psychological health, quality of life, and physical health of patients with cancer: a meta-analysis. Evid Based Complement Alternat Med. 2011;2011:659876.

35. Moadel AB, Shah C, Wylie-Rosett J, et al. Randomized controlled trial of yoga among a multiethnic sample of breast cancer patients: effects on quality of life. J Clin Oncol. 2007;25:4387–95.

36. Danhauer SC, Mihalko SL, Russell GB, et al. Restorative yoga for women with breast cancer: findings from a randomized pilot study. Psychooncology. 2009;18:360–8.

37. Cohen L, Warneke C, Fouladi RT, Rodriguez MA, Chaoul-Reich A. Psychological adjustment and sleep quality in a randomized trial of the effects of a Tibetan yoga intervention in patients with lymphoma. Cancer. 2004;100:2253–60.

38. Buffart L, va Uffelen J, Riphagen I, et al. Physical and psychosocial benefits of yoga in cancer patients and survivors, a systematic review and meta-analysis of randomized controlled trials. BMC Cancer. 2012;12:559.

39. Bower JE, Garet D, Sternlieb B, et al. Yoga for persistent fatigue in breast cancer survivors: a randomized controlled trial. Cancer. 2012; 118:3766–75.

40. McNeely ML, Courneya KS. Exercise programs for cancer-related fatigue: evidence and clinical guidelines. J Natl Compr Canc Netw. 2010;8:945–53.

41. Dimeo FC. Effects of exercise on cancer-related fatigue. Cancer. 2001; 92:1689–93.

42. Schmitz KH, Courneya KS, Matthews C, et al. American college of sports medicine roundtable on exercise guidelines for cancer survivors. Med Sci Sports Exerc. 2010;42:1409–26.

43. Courneya KS. Exercise in cancer survivors: an overview of research. Med Sci Sports Exerc. 2003;35:1846–52.

44. Cramp F, Daniel J. Exercise for the management of cancer-related fatigue in adults. Cochrane Database Syst Rev. 2008:CD006145.

45. Brown JC, Huedo-Medina TB, Pescatello LS, Pescatello SM, Ferrer RA, Johnson BT. Efficacy of exercise interventions in modulating cancer-related fatigue among adult cancer survivors: a meta-analysis. Cancer Epidemiol Biomarkers Prev. 2011;20:123–33.

46. Speck RM, Courneya KS, Masse LC, Duval S, Schmitz KH. An update of controlled physical activity trials in cancer survivors: a systematic review and meta-analysis. J Cancer Surviv. 2010;4:87–100.
47. National Comprehensive Cancer Network (NCCN). Clinical practice guidelines in oncology: cancer related fatigue. Version 1. 2014. www.nccn. org/professionals/physician_gls/pdf/fatigue.pdf. Accessed 25 September 2014.
48. Blaney J, Lowe-Strong A, Rankin J, Campbell A, Allen J, Gracey J. The cancer rehabilitation journey: barriers to and facilitators of exercise among patients with cancer-related fatigue. Phys Ther. 2010;90: 1135–47.

# Chapter 5
# Pharmacological Treatment

## 5.1 Introduction

Pharmacological treatment of cancer-related fatigue (CrF) is generally based on addressing symptoms and reducing intensifying factors such as anemia, malnutrition, sleep, and endocrine disorders, as well as impacting possible pathophysiological factors such as changes in the serotonergic system of the central nervous system (CNS) and dysregulation of inflammatory cytokines. Therefore, medications with a very wide range of mechanisms of action are used to treat CrF [1]. Pharmacologic agents to treat CrF should be used in a conservative manner, especially as many types of treatment are still regarded as experimental therapies that may require more research to prove their safety and efficacy [2].

To date, clinical studies have been carried out on psychostimulants, hematopoietic growth factors, antidepressants, anti-inflammatory drugs including corticosteroids, and phytotherapeutic agents [3]. Regardless of the treatment, if a pharmacological approach is being considered, it should be part of a comprehensive treatment and care plan which is based on the individual and takes into account the extent of functional

J. Weis, M. Horneber, *Cancer-Related Fatigue*,
DOI 10.1007/978-1-907673-76-4_5,
© Springer Healthcare 2015

impairment caused by physical, psychological, and cognitive problems. The clinical and therapeutic prognosis and treatment of the tumor should also be taken into consideration, as should the preferences of the patient [4]. In principle, CrF should be treated as early as possible, as this can prevent fatigue from becoming a chronic condition. This particularly applies when the fatigue symptoms appear before cancer diagnosis and treatment [5].

## 5.2  Stimulants

The National Comprehensive Cancer Network (NCCN) clinical guidelines recommend the use of psychostimulants in CrF [6]. However, recent studies have cast doubt on such broad recommendations, as the beneficial effects of stimulants may be restricted to a specific subgroup of patients [7, 8]. This can be understood from a pathophysiological perspective, as psychostimulants have little effect on inflammatory processes and disorders in the hypothalamic-pituitary adrenal system, which are probable contributing factors to CrF. Given the current clinical data, the use of psychostimulants could be considered for individual patients with severe forms of CrF in whom other treatments have not been successful [7, 8].

### 5.2.1  Methylphenidate

Methylphenidate is an amphetamine that is used off-label for treating CrF. The inhibition of the reuptake of noradrenalin and dopamine from the synaptic gap and an associated increase in sympathetic CNS activity may be a possible pharmacological mechanism of action, as may the effect of methylphenidate as a serotonin receptor antagonist. Dexmethylphenidate, one of the enantiomers of methylphenidate, is also available but neither drug has been specifically approved and marketed for CrF.

A meta-analysis of four trials suggested that methylphenidate may be beneficial for patients with cancer and CrF [9]. A post-hoc analysis of one of the included trials found that patients with higher levels of baseline fatigue appeared to have a better response and that improvement after the first day of treatment with methylphenidate was predictive for long-term improvement [10]. However, results from two large trials found no evidence that methylphenidate is effective in the management of CrF [7, 11]. Although a recent editorial concluded that the evidence against methylphenidate is beginning to accumulate, more research needs to be done to determine efficacy and safety. Undesirable side effects such as nervousness, sleeplessness, headaches, xerostomia, and nausea should be taken into consideration [12].

It should be noted that methylphenidate is a controlled substance with a potential risk of addiction and should be given under strict supervision. Contraindications such as poorly managed arterial hypertension, symptomatic coronary cardiovascular diseases, arrhythmias, and convulsion disorders should also be taken into consideration with methylphenidate use.

## 5.2.2 Modafinil

Modafinil has an effect on various CNS neurotransmitters and can improve consciousness, attention, and motor activity. However, the exact mechanism of action of modafinil is not known and it appears to differ from other psychostimulants from a pharmacological perspective. Modafinil increases hypothalamic histamine levels (much like an amphetamine-like stimulant), while inhibiting the actions of the dopamine transporter.

An improvement in the sleep-wake rhythm is also thought to be a possible mechanism of action.

A meta-analysis by Cooper et al. suggested that modafinil improves CrF in patients who have received cancer treatment, including improvements in cognitive function, general activities (e.g., walking ability, socializing), and enjoyment of life [13]. However, many of the studies included were open-label and uncontrolled, making true clinical significance difficult to determine. In two Phase III, randomized, controlled, double-blind trials, the effect of modafinil was found to be greater than placebo in patients with high baseline, severe forms of CrF ($P = 0.033$) [14]. However, there were no significant differences found between placebo and patients with mild or moderate fatigue (as defined by the Brief Fatigue Inventory). In a recent randomized placebo-controlled trial, no significantly superior effect of modafinil was found when compared to placebo for managing fatigue in lung cancer [15].

In terms of safety, in 2011, the European Medicines Agency (EMA) recommended vigilance with the use of this drug, as modafinil was associated with adverse reactions including hypersensitivity and serious skin reactions (e.g., Stevens Johnson syndrome), neuropsychiatric, and cardiovascular reactions [16]. Safety and efficacy in children has not been established and pediatric use is not recommended.

## 5.3    Erythropoiesis-Stimulating Agents

During chemotherapy, CrF in patients with anemia can be reduced with the use of erythropoiesis-stimulating agents (ESAs) such as epoetin and darbepoetin, although significant improvement was most likely to be seen in patients with at lower hemoglobin concentrations (8–10 g/100 ml) [17]. It is important to note that the majority of patients affected by CrF do not have anemia [18, 19], and their physical capacity is influenced by several other factors such as endothelial function and mitochondria thickness in the muscles. Therefore, the performance of the patients with cancer can be considerably reduced despite normal hemoglobin levels. As such, the use of ESAs should not be based on a target hemoglobin value, but rather on the symptoms and signs of anemia and their impact on physical functioning and other measures of quality of life [20]. A recent meta-analysis of individual patient data from 53 trials revealed an increase in mortality when ESAs were given during chemotherapy (combined hazard ratio = 1.17; 95 % CI, 1.06–1.30) [21], and a higher incidence of thrombotic and thromboembolic events as a result of treatment with ESAs. This data underscore the need for a critical assessment of the benefits and risks of treatment of CrF with ESAs in accordance with current guidelines [20].

## 5.4 Antidepressants

Clinical studies with selective serotonin reuptake inhibitors (SSRIs) have not shown any specific effectiveness on CrF to date and, thus, SSRIs are only a treatment option if the patient is diagnosed with a comorbid depressive disorder [17]. Preliminary evidence suggests that another type of antidepressant, bupropion, a selective norepinephrine-dopamine reuptake inhibitor (NDRI), may be effective in the management of CrF. However, in the absence of data from randomized controlled trials, the evidence should be regarded as tentative and provisional [22, 23].

## 5.5 Corticosteroids

Synthetic glucocorticoids can have positive effects on CrF in palliative care and terminally ill patients with cancer due to their actions on the CNS and on chronic inflammation [24]. A recent trial found a significant improvement of CrF in patients with advanced cancer after 2 weeks of oral dexamethasone [25] and Bruera et al. reported in 1985 an increase in daily activities in terminally ill cancer patients after 4 weeks of methylprednisone [26].

The European Association for Palliative Care recommends short-term use of corticosteroids in palliative care, in particular where CrF is associated with signs and symptoms of anorexia-cachexia syndrome and bone or brain metastases, but it likewise points to the undesirable side effects such as myopathy, depression, and sleep disorders which could increase symptoms associated with CrF [27].

## 5.6  Thyrotropin-Releasing Hormone

Apart from its endocrine properties, thyrotropin-releasing hormone (TRH) is thought to be involved in the restoration of homeostasis of behavioral, metabolic, and immunological processes, which are believed to be related to CrF [28]. The results of a pilot, randomized, placebo-controlled study suggested that the intravenous administration of TRH may be a safe and effective treatment option for CrF. In this study, TRH resulted in an improvement in the symptoms of fatigue, which started a few hours after treatment and continued for several days [29]. However, due to its pharmaceutical properties, TRH analogs with longer plasma half-life, better intestinal and CNS permeability, and lower endocrine activity are being developed.

## 5.7 Phytotherapeutic Agents

### 5.7.1 Ginseng

Ginseng, the root from *Panax* species, is a traditional herbal remedy used to treat all kinds of fatigue. Ginsenosides are the putative main active compounds and are nearly exclusively found in *Panax* species. The content of ginsenosides is seen as a measurement of the quality of a ginseng root. Preferably, the plant is harvested once at 4–7 years old and all parts of the root (primary root, lateral roots and rootlets including their peel) are processed [30]. The affinity of ginsenosides for glucocorticoid receptors, their effect on stress-induced neuronal activity, inflammatory mediators, and their membrane-stabilizing effects are all considered as a possible basis for the pharmacological effects in fatigue [31, 32].

In clinical studies on CrF, the American ginseng (*Panax quinquefolius*) and the Asian ginseng (*Panax ginseng* C.A. Meyer) were investigated [33, 34]. The results of the studies suggest that both extracts of *Panax quinquefolius* and of *Panax ginseng* can effectively reduce CrF. For example, in a multicenter, randomized, double blind, placebo-controlled study 364 patients with at least moderate fatigue received 2,000 mg of American ginseng or placebo for 8 weeks. Changes in fatigue, as measured by the Multidimensional Fatigue Symptom Inventory-Short Form (MFSI-SF), from baseline to 4 and 8 weeks were 14.4 and 20, respectively, in the ginseng group compared to 8.2 and 10.3 in the placebo group. Additionally, patients who were on active cancer treatment perceived greater benefit [35].

In some countries (e.g., Germany), preparations of *P. ginseng* are approved drugs to treat fatigue [36]. Preparations of

*P. ginseng* and *P. quinquefolius* are usually well tolerated with only minor and easily reversible undesirable effects including headaches, sleep disturbances and gastrointestinal intolerance [37, 38].

## 5.7.2  Guarana *(Paullinia cupana)*

Indications for the effectiveness of guarana (*Paullinia cupana*) come from a clinical study in which guarana improved CrF during chemotherapy in 75 patients with breast cancer [39]. In the study, patients with progressive fatigue following the first cycle of chemotherapy were randomized to receive either guarana 50 mg twice-daily or placebo, crossing over half-way through the study. Guarana was found to significantly improve Functional Assessment of Chronic Illness Therapy-Fatigue (FACIT-F), Functional Assessment of Chronic Illness Therapy-Endocrine Symptoms (FACT-ES), and Brief Fatigue Inventory global scores when compared to placebo ($P<0.01$) [39]. An earlier trial of the same group, however, found no beneficial effects of guarana on the the incidence and severity of CrF during radiotherapy [40]. The main active ingredient of guarana is caffeine, which is released more slowly than from coffee [41]. The amount of guarana administered in the studies contains approximately one-tenth the amount in a cup of coffee.

## 5.7.3  Other Herbal Drugs

There is preliminary evidence from randomized trials of beneficial effects concerning symptoms of fatigue come from other herbal extracts such as tragacanth (*Astragalus membranaceus*) for CrF [42], roseroot (*Rhodiola rosea*) for stress-related fatigue [43], valerian (*Valeriana* L.) for CrF [44], and magnolia vine (*Schisandra chinensis*) for cognitive fatigue [45].

# References

1. Bruera E, Yennurajalingam S. Challenge of managing cancer-related fatigue. J Clin Oncol. 2010;28:3671–2.
2. Howell D, Keller-Olaman S, Oliver TK, et al. A pan-Canadian practice guideline and algorithm: screening, assessment, and supportive care of adults with cancer-related fatigue. Curr Oncol. 2013;20:e233–46.
3. Bower JE. Treating cancer-related fatigue: the search for interventions that target those most in need. J Clin Oncol. 2012;30:4449–50.
4. Horneber M, Fischer I, Dimeo F, Ruffer JU, Weis J. Cancer-related fatigue: epidemiology, pathogenesis, diagnosis, and treatment. Dtsch Arztebl Int. 2012;109:161–71.
5. Kuhnt S, Ehrensperger C, Singer S, et al. Prädiktoren tumorassoziierter fatigue. Psychotherapeut. 2011;56:216–23.
6. National Comprehensive Cancer Network (NCCN). Cancer-related fatigue. NCCN clinical practice guidelines in oncology. Version 1. 2014. www.nccn.org/professionals/physician_gls/f_guidelines.asp. Accessed 25 September 2014.
7. Bruera E, Yennurajalingham S, Palmer JL, et al. Methylphenidate and/or a nursing telephone intervention for fatigue in patients with advanced cancer: A randomized, placebo-controlled, phase II trial. J Clin Oncol. 2013;31:2421–7.
8. Fife K, Spathis A, Dutton SJ, et al. A multicenter, randomized, double-blinded, placebo-controlled trial of modafinil for lung cancer-related fatigue: dose response and patient satisfaction data. J Clin Oncol. 2013;31(Suppl):9503.
9. Minton O, Richardson A, Sharpe M, Hotopf M, Stone PC. Psychostimulants for the management of cancer-related fatigue: a systematic review and meta-analysis. J Pain Symptom Manage. 2011;41:761–7.
10. Yennurajalingam S, Palmer JL, Chacko R, Bruera E. Factors associated with response to methylphenidate in advanced cancer patients. Oncologist. 2011;16:246–53.
11. Moraska AR, Sood A, Dakhil SR, et al. Phase III, randomized, double-blind, placebo-controlled study of long-acting methylphenidate for cancer-related fatigue: North Central Cancer Treatment Group NCCTG-N05C7 Trial. J Clin Oncol. 2010;28:3673–9.
12. Stone PC. Methylphenidate in the management of cancer-related fatigue. J Clin Oncol. 2013;31:2372–3.
13. Cooper MR, Bird HM, Steinberg M. Efficacy and safety of modafinil in the treatment of cancer-related fatigue. Ann Pharmacother. 2009;43:721–5.

14. Jean-Pierre P, Morrow GR, Roscoe JA, et al. A Phase 3 randomized, placebo-controlled, double-blind, clinical trial of the effect of modafinil on cancer-related fatigue among 631 patients receiving chemotherapy. Cancer. 2010;15:3513–20.

15. Spathis A, Fife K, Blackhall F, et al. Modafinil for the treatment of fatigue in lung cancer: results of a placebo-controlled, double-blind, randomized trial. J Clin Oncol. 2014;32:1882–8.

16. European Medicines Agency (EMA). Assessment report for modafinil containing medicinal products. www.ema.europa.eu/docs/en_GB/document_library/Referrals_document/Modafinil_31/WC500105597.pdf. Accessed 25 September 2014.

17. Minton O, Stone P, Richardson A, Sharpe M, Hotopf M. Drug therapy for the management of cancer related fatigue. Cochrane Database Syst Rev. 2010;(7):CD006704.

18. Dimeo F, Schmittel A, Fietz T, et al. Physical performance, depression, immune status and fatigue in patients with hematological malignancies after treatment. Ann Oncol. 2004;15:1237–42.

19. Geinitz H, Zimmermann FB, Stoll P, et al. Fatigue, serum cytokine levels, and blood cell counts during radiotherapy of patients with breast cancer. Int J Radiat Oncol Biol Phys. 2001;51:691–8.

20. Rizzo JD, Brouwers M, Hurley P, et al. American Society of Clinical Oncology/American Society of Hematology clinical practice guideline update on the use of epoetin and darbepoetin in adult patients with cancer. J Clin Oncol. 2010;28:4996–5010.

21. Bohlius J, Schmidlin K, Brillant C, et al. Recombinant human erythropoiesis-stimulating agents and mortality in patients with cancer: a meta-analysis of randomised trials. Lancet.009;373:1532–42.

22. Moss EL, Simpson JS, Pelletier G, Forsyth P. An open-label study of the effects of bupropion SR on fatigue, depression and quality of life of mixed-site cancer patients and their partners. Psychooncology. 2006;15:259–67.

23. Cullum JL, Wojciechowski AE, Pelletier G, Simpson JS. Bupropion sustained release treatment reduces fatigue in cancer patients. Can J Psychiatry. 2004;49:139–44.

24. Shih A, Jackson KC. Role of corticosteroids in palliative care. J Pain Palliat Care Pharmacother. 2007;21:69–76.

25. Yennurajalingam S, Frisbee-Hume S, Palmer JL, et al. Reduction of cancer-related fatigue with dexamethasone: a double-blind, randomized, placebo-controlled trial in patients with advanced cancer. J Clin Oncol. 2013;31:3076–82.

26. Bruera E, Roca E, Cedaro L, et al. Action of oral methylprednisolone in terminal cancer patients: a prospective randomized double-blind study. Cancer Treat Rep. 1985;69:751–4.

27. Radbruch L, Strasser F, Elsner F, et al. Fatigue in palliative care patients - an EAPC approach. Palliat Med. 2008;22:13–32.

28. Kamath J, Yarbrough GG, Prange Jr AJ, Winokur A. The thyrotropin-releasing hormone (TRH)-immune system homeostatic hypothesis. Pharmacol Ther. 2009;121:20–8.

29. Kamath J, Feinn R, Winokur A. Thyrotropin-releasing hormone as a treatment for cancer-related fatigue: a randomized controlled study. Support Care Cancer. 2012;20:1745–53.

30. Choi KT. Botanical characteristics, pharmacological effects and medicinal components of Korean Panax ginseng C A Meyer. Acta Pharmacol Sin. 2008;29:1109–18.

31. Rasheed N, Tyagi E, Ahmad A, Siripurapu KB, Lahiri S, Shukla R, Palit G. Involvement of monoamines and proinflammatory cytokines in mediating the anti-stress effects of Panax quinquefolium. J Ethnopharmacol. 2008;117:257–62.

32. Radad K, Moldzio R, Rausch WD. Ginsenosides and their CNS targets. CNS Neurosci Ther. 2011;17:761–8.

33. Lee NH, Son CG. Systematic review of randomized controlled trials evaluating the efficacy and safety of ginseng. J Acupunct Meridian Stud. 2011;4:85–97.

34. Finnegan-John J, Molassiotis A, Richardson A, Ream E. A systematic review of complementary and alternative medicine interventions for the management of cancer-related fatigue. Integr Cancer Ther. 2013;12:276–90.

35. Barton DL, Liu H, Dakhil SR, et al. Wisconsin Ginseng (Panax quinquefolius) to improve cancer-related fatigue: a randomized, Double-Blind Trial, N07C2. J Natl Cancer Inst. 2013;105:1230–8.

36. World Health Organization (WHO). WHO monographs on medicinal plants commonly use in the newly independent states. Geneva: WHO Press; 2010.

37. Kitts DD, Hu C. Efficacy and safety of ginseng. Public Health Nutr. 2000;34:473–85.

38. Coon JT, Ernst E. Panax ginseng: a systematic review of adverse effects and drug interactions. Drug Saf. 2002;25:323–44.

39. Campos MP, Riechelmann R, Martins LC, Hassan BJ, Casa FB, Del Giglio A. Effect of guarana (Paullinia cupana) on fatigue in breast cancer patients undergoing systemic chemotherapy. J Clin Oncol. 2010;28:9007.

40. da Costa Miranda V, Trufelli DC, Santos J, et al. Effectiveness of guarana (*Paullinia cupana*) for postradiation fatigue and depression: results of a pilot double-blind randomized study. J Altern Complement Med. 2009;15:431–3.
41. Haensel R, Pertz H. Alkaloide. In: Hänsel R, Sticher O, editors. Pharmakognosie phytopharmazie. Heidelberg: Springer Medizin; 2007:1455–6.
42. Chen HW, Lin IH, Chen YJ, et al. A novel infusible botanically-derived drug, PG2, for cancer-related fatigue: a phase II double-blind, randomized placebo-controlled study. Clin Invest Med. 2012;35:E1–11.
43. Olsson EM, von Schéele B, Panossian AG. A randomised, double-blind, placebo-controlled, parallel-group study of the standardised extract shr-5 of the roots of Rhodiola rosea in the treatment of subjects with stress-related fatigue. Planta Med. 2009;75:105–12.
44. Barton DL, Atherton PJ, Bauer BA, et al. The use of Valeriana officinalis (Valerian) in improving sleep in patients who are undergoing treatment for cancer: a phase III randomized, placebo-controlled, double-blind study (NCCTG Trial, N01C5). J Support Oncol. 2011;9: 24–31.
45. Aslanyan G, Amroyan E, Gabrielyan E, Nylander M, Wikman G, Panossian A. Double-blind, placebo-controlled, randomised study of single dose effects of ADAPT-232 on cognitive functions. Phytomedicine. 2010;17:494–9.

# Chapter 6
# Recommendations for the Management of Cancer-Related Fatigue

## 6.1 Introduction

Despite being one of the most common symptoms associated with cancer, studies have shown that patient complaints and symptoms of cancer-related fatigue (CrF) are often overlooked, with 80 % of oncologists believing that it is undertreated [1]. Reasons for insufficient communication around CrF lie both with patients affected with CrF as well as health care providers. This may be due to the fact that fatigue can be notoriously hard to define, as it arises from an unpredictable interplay of physical and psychological factors, which patients may simply accept as 'part of the disease' [2]. Additionally, health care providers may not accurately perceive the magnitude of the stresses and restrictions caused by CrF to a sufficient extent and underestimate treatment needs [3].

Following cancer treatment, patients may also fear that fatigue is a sign of recurrence of the illness or that further treatment could be delayed [4, 5]. The most frequently reported reasons for lack of patient communication about fatigue include the doctor's failure to offer interventions, patients' lack of awareness of effective treatments, patient preferring to treat fatigue without

J. Weis, M. Horneber, *Cancer-Related Fatigue*,
DOI 10.1007/978-1-907673-76-4_6,
© Springer Healthcare 2015

medication, and the patient not wanting to complain to the doctor [6]. Additionally, people close to the patient are also affected, as CrF can have an impact on family roles, often leaving both patients and their families struggling to cope [7].

## 6.2  Screening and Assessment

Against this background, fatigue should be systematically assessed by a stepped diagnostic strategy, starting with a screening procedure to identify the level of fatigue. According to the guidelines of the Canadian Association of Psychosocial Oncology and the National Comprehensive Cancer Network (NCCN), patients with cancer should be asked directly about CrF at regular intervals during treatment and follow-up using a self-rating scale [8, 9]. The use of a visual or linear analog scale has been proven to be an effective instrument to identify the intensity of fatigue [10, 11]. Based on this scale, scores ranging from 0 to 3 are interpreted as mild fatigue, 4–6 as moderate, and 7–10 as severe fatigue. A reported intensity of $\geq 4$ is the threshold value for further diagnostic assessments which should include a thorough history of fatigue and possible contributing risk factors (e.g., depression, anemia, pain, nausea, sleep disturbance, comorbidities), a physical examination and a self-assessment of causes contributing to fatigue. Assessments should be a shared responsibility of an expert clinical team [8].

The various psychological factors influencing CrF should be assessed by clinical interviews, including psychological distress, anxiety, depression, and sleeping disorders. Many patients initially react to CrF with a 'fighting spirit' and positive thinking; however, dejection and disappointment can set in if the fatigue persists and strength continuously decreases [12, 13]. Many of those affected with fatigue also suffer from pain, sleep disorders, and psychological stress due to anxiety and depression [14, 15]. Somatic comorbidities such as cardiovascular, pulmonary, renal, hepatic, or neurologic dysfunction should be assessed by clinical examination. Aside from cancer and its treatment, these dysfunctions may be potential causes of the fatigue symptoms, although in clinical practice it is often difficult to differentiate between fatigue due to comorbidities and fatigue caused by cancer and/or cancer treatment. Lab parameters (e.g., blood counts, thyroid-stimulating hormone [TSH], electrolytes, glucose, transaminases) should be assessed. If there is any evidence of dysfunction, causal therapy should be recommended as the first step of fatigue management.

Aside from cancer treatments, fatigue is a frequent side effect of other drug therapies commonly used alongside cancer therapies for often unrelated comorbidities (e.g., mood disorders, allergies). Some drugs may result in an imbalance between inhibitory and excitatory pathways in the CNS, which can lead to a so-called 'central fatigue' [16].

**Opioids** can cause fatigue and sedation, regardless of dosing or strength. While sedation is a symptom of overdose, fatigue (as well as nausea, vomiting), mostly disappears during the first two weeks of treatment.

**Benzodiazepines** with a long half-life or active metabolites may lead to a sedative effect. An example can be seen with tetrazepam, a centrally-acting muscle relaxant.

**Tricyclic antidepressants** have known anticholinergic and sedative effects. The latter are more pronounced for amitriptyline and doxepine than for the other antidepressants.

**Antipsychotic drugs** such as low potency antipsychotic drugs cause sedation (e.g., levomepromazine, melperone, pipamperone). Even newer antipsychotic drugs such as olanzapine and clozapine cause fatigue in up to 40 % of patients.

**Antihypertensive drugs**, such as clonidine and moxonidine, as well as alpha-blockers, beta-blockers, and angiotensin-converting-enzyme (ACE) inhibitors can cause fatigue. Within the group of beta-blockers, the lipophilic substances that can better penetrate into the CNS, for example propranolol, cause fatigue more frequently, this can, however, also be caused by beta-blocker-induced sleep disorder.

**Second-generation antihistamines** such as loratadine, fexofenadine, cetirizine have less sedative effects than first-generation agents (diphenhydramine, dimenhydrinate, dimetindene), which are also used for mild sedation [17].

The history, in combination with the physical examination, can provide clues to possible causes or contributing factors. If the history, physical examination, and basic laboratory tests yield no evidence of any underlying functional disturbance, further laboratory testing and technical examinations are generally of little use and should only be performed if the basic diagnostic assessment yielded unequivocally abnormal findings. If allocation of the symptoms to a diagnosis is not (unambiguously) possible, great care should be taken so that diagnostic associations or suspected diagnoses do not contain any unsubstantiated prejudices. This is important because causal implications may be concluded, and physical symptoms may falsely appear as a manifestation of psychological disorder or fixation on physiological causes impedes to take psychological factors into consideration.

## 6.3    Information and Counseling

Regardless of the screening method and diagnostic procedures, core information and counseling should be offered to all patients, which can be through the use of brochures, written material, or web-based information. For patients with a fatigue score over the diagnostic threshold, further assessment and individual counseling are recommended to identify potential influencing factors. Generally, supportive interventions such as exercise or psychosocial interventions may be helpful for patients at all levels of fatigue, provided that the physical performance status of the patients allows such activities. For patients with severe CrF (visual analog score [VAS] $\geq 7$), additional pharmacological treatment of CRF might be considered if other potential

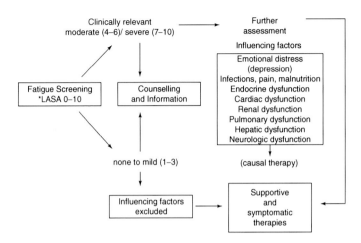

**Fig. 6.1** Algorithm for the assessment of cancer-related fatigue according to the NCCN guidelines. LASA, linear analog self-assessment. (Reproduced with permission from NCCN [9] ©National Comprehensive Cancer Network)

influencing factors of fatigue have been ruled out (see Chaps. 4 and 5 for more information about treatment options). The algorithm in Fig. 6.1 summarizes the process of assessment based on the multi-modal approach. Based on this algorithm, patients should be treated according to when CrF occurs. When planning supportive interventions, a stepped care approach is recommended. Generally, evidenced-based treatment strategies should be selected according to the patient's needs and preferences.

## 6.4   Cancer-Related Fatigue During Cancer Treatment

Signs and symptoms of CrF may start during chemotherapy, radiotherapy, and/or hormone therapy and continue over a certain time after the treatment has been completed [18, 19]. As such forms of treatment-associated CrF are regarded as a risk factor for developing persisting CrF, it is recommended to provide the patient with information about CrF and/or provide individual counseling as early as possible. Practicing the general strategies for managing fatigue such as monitoring fatigue, energy conservation, setting priorities, pacing regular activities and distraction help the patient to cope better with CrF and may prevent persisting CrF [8].

With individual counseling, it is also important to inform and encourage the patient that there is a high probability that CrF will continuously decrease after the end of treatment. This information could influence the patient's understanding of and attitude towards their fatigue symptoms. In addition, treatment approaches such as exercise, psychosocial and mind-body interventions and acupuncture should be recommended for the patients during and immediately after cancer treatment as part of a comprehensive concept of supportive care for managing treatment-associated side effects (see Chaps. 4 and 5) [8].

## 6.5   Persisting Cancer-Related Fatigue

As discussed above, CrF can persist or recur as a long-term sequelae for many years once anticancer and antineoplastic treatment has ceased [20–23]. In those cases when CrF has persisted over time or has recurred after a period of relatively good health, the interpretation to what extent fatigue is directly associated with cancer or its treatment is often difficult and most widely unclear. Long-term fatigue may be influenced by the adjustment to the altered health conditions and, therefore, interfered by more or less adaptive or maladaptive emotions and cognitions of the patients. This could be also interpreted as a response to various types of experienced distress of survivors such as a fear of recurrence or fear of progression. Thus, potential somatic late effects of cancer treatment (e.g., cardio-myopathy) should be checked before planning any individual treatment.

Following the NCCN algorithm (Fig. 6.1) and the recommendations of the current Canadian practice guideline, after examination of potential somatic factors and late effects as potential causes of fatigue, psychosocial interventions such as cognitive behavioral techniques (CBT) and psychoeducational approaches are adequate strategies for changing maladaptive thoughts and supporting the patient's management of fatigue [8, 9]. Regular activities and exercise could be combined with psychosocial and mind-body interventions to improve the symptoms of fatigue.

Pharmacological treatment should be used only if other treatment approaches have not shown any effects and high levels of fatigue are still ongoing [24]. In the absence of robust evidence, decisions about whether pharmacologic agents are likely to be beneficial for a particular situation should rely on expert judgment and practical considerations.

## 6.6 Fatigue in the Palliative Situation

In palliative care settings, CrF is often combined with multiple other symptoms such as dyspnea, pain, and cachexia [25, 26]. Therefore, the management of CrF should include thorough symptom management as part of a comprehensive palliative care approach [27]. As a major part of this approach, the individual preferences and needs of the patient have to be considered and the trade-offs between advantages and disadvantages of CrF treatment should be discussed with the multidisciplinary palliative care team [28]. Following the results of a recent trial, dexamethasone was found to be effective for a temporary relief in cases of severe fatigue in the palliative care setting [29].

# References

1. Vogelzang NJ, Breitbart W, Cella D, et al. Patient, caregiver, and oncologist perceptions of cancer-related fatigue. Results of a Tripart assessment survey. Semin Hematol. 1997;34 Suppl 2:4–12.
2. Pearce S, Richardson A. Fatigue in cancer: a phenomenological perspective. Eur J Cancer Care (Engl). 1996;5:111–5.
3. Newell S, Sanson-Fisher RW, Girgis A, Bonaventura A. How well do medical oncologists' perceptions reflect their patients' reported physical and psychosocial problems? Data from a survey of five oncologists. Cancer. 1998;83:1640–51.
4. Shun SC, Lai YH, Hsiao FH. Patient-related barriers to fatigue communication in cancer patients receiving active treatment. Oncologist. 2009;14:936–43.
5. Westerman MJ, The AM, Sprangers MA, Groen HJ, van der Wal G, Hak T. Small-cell lung cancer patients are just 'a little bit' tired: response shift and self-presentation in the measurement of fatigue. Qual Life Res. 2007;16:853–61.
6. Passik SD, Kirsh KL, Donaghy K, et al. Patient-related barriers to fatigue communication: initial validation of the fatigue management barriers questionnaire. J Pain Symptom Manage. 2002;24:481–93.
7. Oktay JS, Bellin MH, Scarvalone S, Appling S, Helzlsouer KJ. Managing the impact of posttreatment fatigue on the family: breast cancer survivors share their experiences. Fam Syst Health. 2011;29: 127–37.
8. Howell D, Keller-Olaman S, Oliver TK, et al. A pan-Canadian practice guideline and algorithm: screening, assessment, and supportive care of adults with cancer-related fatigue. Curr Oncol. 2013;20:e233–46.
9. National Comprehensive Cancer Network (NCCN). Clinical practice guidelines in oncology: cancer related fatigue. Version 1. 2014. www.nccn. org/professionals/physician_gls/pdf/fatigue.pdf. Accessed 25 September 2014.
10. Given B, Given CW, Sikorskii A, et al. Establishing mild, moderate, and severe scores for cancer-related symptoms: how consistent and clinically meaningful are interference-based severity cutpoints? J Pain Symptom Manage. 2008;35:126–35.
11. Butt Z, Wagner LI, Beaumont JL. Use of a single item screening instrument to detect clinically relevant fatigue, distress, pain and anorexia in ambulatory cancer practice. J Pain Symptom Manage. 2008;35: 20–30.

12. Shi Q, Smith TG, Michonski JD, Stein KD, Kaw C, Cleeland CS. Symptom burden in cancer survivors 1 year after diagnosis: a report from the American Cancer Society's studies of cancer survivors. Cancer. 2011;117:2779–90.

13. Scott JA, Lasch KE, Barsevick AM, Piault-Louis E. Patients' experiences with cancer-related fatigue: a review and synthesis of qualitative research. Oncol Nurs Forum. 2011;38:E191–203.

14. Brown LF, Kroenke K. Cancer-related fatigue and its associations with depression and anxiety: a systematic review. Psychosomatics. 2009;50: 440–7.

15. Ancoli-Israel S, Moore PJ, Jones V. The relationship between fatigue and sleep in cancer patients: a review. Eur J Cancer Care (Engl). 2001; 10:245–55.

16. Zlott DA, Byrne M. Mechanisms by which pharmacologic agents may contribute to fatigue. PMR. 2010;2:451–5.

17. Brunton L, Chabner B, Knollman B. Goodman and Gilman's the pharmacological basis of therapeutics. 12th ed. New York: McGraw Hill; 2011.

18. Meraner V, Gamper EM, Grahmann A. Monitoring physical and psychosocial symptom trajectories in ovarian cancer patients receiving chemotherapy. BMC Cancer. 2012;12:77.

19. Ameringer S, Elswick Jr RK, Shockey DP, Dillon R. A pilot exploration of symptom trajectories in adolescents with cancer during chemotherapy. Cancer Nurs. 2013;36:60–71.

20. Rueffer JU, Flechtner H, Tralls P, et al. Fatigue in long-term survivors of Hodgkin's lymphoma; a report from the German Hodgkin Lymphoma Study Group (GHSG). Eur J Cancer. 2003;39:2179–86.

21. Berglund G, Boland C, Fornandes T, et al. Late effects of adjuvant chemotherapy and postoperative radiotherapy on quality of life among breast cancer patients. Eur J Cancer. 1991;27:1075–81.

22. Bower J, Ganz P, Desmond K, Rowland J, Meyerowitz B, Belin R. Fatigue in breast cancer survivors: occurrence, correlates, an impact of quality of life. J Clin Oncol. 2000;18:743–53.

23. Servaes P, van-der-Werf S, Prins J, Verhagen S, Bleijenberg G. Fatigue in disease-free cancer patients compared with fatigue in patients with Chronic Fatigue Syndrome. Support Care Cancer. 2001;9:11–7.

24. Horneber M, Fischer I, Dimeo F, Ruffer JU, Weis J. Cancer-related fatigue: epidemiology, pathogenesis, diagnosis, and treatment. Dtsch Arztebl Int. 2012;109:161–71.

25. Yennurajalingam S, Bruera E. Palliative management of fatigue at the close of life: "it feels like my body is just worn out". JAMA. 2007;297: 295–304.

26. Olson K, Krawchuk A, Quddusi T. Fatigue in individuals with advanced cancer in active treatment and palliative settings. Cancer Nurs. 2007;30:E1–10.
27. de Raaf PJ, de Klerk C, Timman R, Busschbach JJ, Oldenmenger WH, van der Rijt CC. Systematic monitoring and treatment of physical symptoms to alleviate fatigue in patients with advanced cancer: a randomized controlled trial. J Clin Oncol. 2013;31:716–23.
28. Radbruch L, Strasser F, Elsner F, et al. Fatigue in palliative care patients – an EAPC approach. Palliat Med. 2008;22:13–32.
29. Yennurajalingam S, Frisbee-Hume S, Palmer JL, et al. Reduction of cancer-related fatigue with dexamethasone: a double-blind, randomized, placebo-controlled trial in patients with advanced cancer. J Clin Oncol. 2013;31:3076–82.

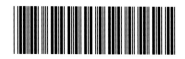